CW00954244

Arthritis:

Escape The Pain

(How I overcame arthritis & how you can too!)

Sarah Woodside

Table of Contents

Introduction: Overcoming The Curse of Arthritis

Living with arthritis isn't easy. It can be excruciatingly painful, cause serious limitations to your mobility, and cause major disruptions to your daily life. You may experience regular bouts of fatigue and exhaustion. You may be unable to work or do the things you love. You may become frustrated, angry, or depressed. Living with arthritis can have a negative effect on your self-esteem, your hope for the future, and your relationships with friends and family.

There are over 200 types of arthritis; most of which can affect you at any age. Your condition may cause pain to one or more specific joints due to a past injury or repetitive strain or it may be a systemic condition causing inflammation throughout your entire body. Depending on the type of arthritis you suffer from, your doctor may prescribe daily medication or painkillers to take as needed. Anti-inflammatories (both prescription and those bought over the counter) can provide significant pain relief, but there are many other ways you can reduce your pain and increase your mobility. *When it comes to treating arthritis, there are far more options than you might think!*

This book does not claim to give you a life-long complete 100% *cure* for arthritis; nor will it ever encourage you to stop taking medicines prescribed by your doctor. Any book that makes these claims is frankly trying to scam you. Rather, in this book I will show you how I overcame my dark days living with rheumatoid arthritis through natural means. I will offer you a variety of natural treatments including making changes to your diet, effectively taking nutritional supplements, creating an appropriate balance of rest and exercise, and maintaining a positive, hopeful attitude. There are many things you can do to ensure better mobility, significantly reduced pain, and an overall healthier, happier life. I will also provide you with a number of practical solutions to common limitations arthritis may cause including accident prevention, making your home an arthritis-friendly place, getting maximum benefits from heat and ice, getting a better quality of sleep, and talking to others about your condition.

My aim is to bring you all the latest developments in dealing with and escaping arthritic pain in a simple to read book, without the non-stop medical jargon. I understand you just want to know how to get better; this book *will* help you!

My Story

I was fifteen years old when my arthritis was discovered for the first time. I was attending the hospital for a bone scan, the purpose of which was to see if I may have had one or more stress fractures in my lower legs. I had been experiencing a lot of pain and naturally, I thought that I must have injured myself. During the bone scan, the doctors looked only at my lower body, as that was where the pain was centered. I doubt anyone was expecting what was found. I know I wasn't.

The doctor called me in and told me that I had signs of early arthritis in every joint from my hips down. My feet and ankles were teeming with what they call "hot spots". My knees and hips were much the same. At the time, I didn't really comprehend what they were saying to me. I didn't have pain in all of my joints. I was very flexible and fit. I remember saying, "Isn't arthritis something that only old people get? I feel FINE!". I was very scared and confused.

After the bone scan, I put everything that happened that day behind me. Apparently I had arthritis, but I didn't feel like anything was wrong. My body wasn't compromised in any way. I didn't understand that what the doctor found in my legs was going to progress, or that it would affect me dramatically later in life. I didn't really understand it at all. So, as any teenager would do, I forgot about it and carried on with my life.

In the few years that followed, I sustained a series of injuries; far more than any of my peers. I had multiple sprains and strains, tendonitis in my ankles and knees, a dislocated collarbone, and a serious injury to my lower back. It was as if my body was more fragile than other people's. There was always *something* that was hurting. But I put all that down to my very active lifestyle. I was a cheerleader at school. I was in dance classes every night and worked as a waitress on the weekends. It seemed likely that all of this activity could perceivably cause my constant state of injury and I never really gave it much thought. Perhaps, I was being naive. After all, how many of us spend our youth thinking about what obstacles we may have to cross in our adulthood? I certainly didn't.

I remember when I started feeling arthritis pain because it actually seemed rather funny, as strange as that sounds! I was eighteen years old and I thought I was having "growing pains". The pain was exactly like those pains I'd had as a small child and I remember joking about how I must've been about to have a growth spurt as an adult!

Indeed, the pain started in my lower body; around those "hot spots" I was once warned about. In the mornings I would wake with a heavy ache in my hips. They felt "full" to me; as if someone had stuffed my joints full of lead. My feet and ankles followed closely behind. I was in my early twenties when I finally consulted my GP. I was in pain regularly and I felt very tired most days, but my blood tests came back inconclusive. The results suggested that I had some inflammation but little else. The GP was wishy-washy about the whole thing. She mentioned something about "mixed connective tissue disease" and hurried me out of the office. Again, I didn't really understand what I was hearing. I thought the GP was suggesting that there wasn't anything wrong with me. And eventually - thinking I must be crazy - I left the whole thing behind me once more, and tried to carry on with my young adult life.

Things progressed much the same for quite a while. I was tired a lot. I had pain and stiffness which I blamed on my previous back injury. My mobility was strange and constantly in flux. I would feel fit as a fiddle one day and then I could barely get out of bed the next. My friends asked me all the time what it was that was wrong with me, my answer to which was plainly, "I don't know".

It was almost a decade later that things really changed for me. I had two children small who I was struggling to keep up with. My tiredness had become full-fledged exhaustion and I found myself in bed most nights before 7pm, too weary to stay up any later. And although my daily pain had increased gradually over the years, the thing that *really* defined the change in my condition was the crippling flare-ups I started experiencing. Days or even weeks would go by where I couldn't get out of bed. My hands were stiff and almost impossible to use. My shoulders curled forward with an ache so intense I could barely lift my arms. Even my jaw would tighten up making it hard to eat or speak. It was like having a really awful flu in my joints. It wasn't long before I was diagnosed with rheumatoid arthritis, and I felt it with the force of a death sentence.

A slue of words coursed through my mind after the official diagnosis, making me feel helpless and hopeless… *progressive… degenerative… limited mobility… no cure*. My spirits plummeted. In all of my anger and frustration, I became depressed and isolated. I gave up on life, spending more and more time in bed. I was eating poorly, drinking too much, and opting out of social events. I had given up my job due to the unpredictable bouts of pain I was feeling so regularly. All I could think about were the things I couldn't do and wouldn't be able to do in the future.

I am happy to say that things did eventually turn around for me and it's a wonderful thing for me to be able to tell this story from a much happier, pain-free future! The big change didn't happen overnight though, and it wasn't easy. The first few years after my diagnosis were pretty terrible. I can say now, looking back, that simply taking medication wasn't enough. I wasn't doing anything to improve my condition or my quality of life. In fact, the way I was living was only contributing to my pain and stiffness. My health was at an all time low. I had gained a ton of weight and I was sick constantly.

It took a lot of research, guidance from my doctor, and personal dedication to overcome that dark period in my life. But slowly, things really improved. I found that there was a lot more I could do to make a difference in my condition and I resolved to do anything I could to make my life better. Taking medicine was helpful, and I would never go against my doctor's wishes where that was concerned, but the *real* lasting changes came from changing my diet (shockingly probably the most important factor), adding exercise into my life, and keeping a positive mental attitude.

My journey to wellness wasn't always easy but it was well worth it. Today, I am happy to report that my rheumatoid arthritis is in remission, where I am absolutely convinced it will remain. I am well enough to work, travel, *and* play with my children. My body is strong enough to fight colds and flus without triggering a flare up. My mobility is better now than it was a decade ago!

I know that there is no absolute *cure* for arthritis and that I will have this condition for the rest of my life. But I also know now that there are ways to overcome it and make living with it easier. You *can* escape the pain. By dedicating myself to my combined mind and body wellness, I have given myself a second chance at life. I am hopeful about my future now and I hope that my story will help and inspire other people living with arthritis to fight back. You don't have to live with all that pain! There are things you can do to make your life better!

Before I go on to tell you how I got where I am today, there is one thing I must stress: I did not go through my journey alone. My doctor was the most valuable resource I had when I set off to improve my condition. With her support and superior knowledge, I was able to successfully pinpoint the things that were triggering my arthritis and safely remove them from my life. My blood levels were tested regularly and I met with her frequently to make sure my health was on the right track. I highly recommend getting guidance from your GP, arthritis specialist, or a well trained dietician in order to ensure safety and success as you embark on your journey.

Let us begin!

Your Experience With Arthritis

Arthritis and other similar inflammatory conditions are different for everyone. Some people experience constant pain, severe problems with mobility, and an inability to carry out normal daily routines. Others may feel only slight discomfort, periodic flare-ups, and on/off joint stiffness. In addition to the differences in each of our conditions, we all have different lives as well. Some people have very demanding careers or home lives. Others may have had to give up work because of the severity of their arthritis. Some people can get by on their own while others need to employ a home care system. Throughout this book, you will see that I regularly refer to *your* condition rather than generalizing arthritic conditions where possible. This is because when treating your arthritis naturally, you must take your particular illness and your life into account rather than comparing yourself to others who have similar conditions. For instance, if you have a fairly busy life and your arthritis is just starting to get in the way of things, you'll need a slightly different care plan than someone who has had to give up work and employ carers because their mobility is so poor. Your condition may be progressing rapidly while others' move more slowly. You may experience flare-ups two or more times per month; others might have just one or two a year. Your medical history is unique to you. Your experience is unique to you. And so your treatment should be unique to you!

In addition, it's important to recognize that some of the treatments in this book will work for you and some may not. There may be certain natural treatments that will not suit your lifestyle or you may not be able to make certain changes to your diet because it may affect another illness like diabetes or high blood pressure. However, no matter who you are or what your life is like, there are plenty of things you can do to make living with your condition easier and it's important to keep an open, positive mind throughout your journey. Natural treatments may not have an *immediate* effect on your condition but they may provide better, longer-lasting relief from daily pain and immobility. They did for me and many other people I talked to when researching this book.

The treatments in this book cover a range of ways you can prevent flare-ups, treat acute pain, slow the progression of your condition, and even put it into remission.

These methods include:

1.) Implementing subtle changes into your life that can help you cope with pain and stiffness.

2.) Diet and exercise regimes that prevent flare-ups, reduce inflammation, and increase mobility.

3.) Practical tips for support and accident prevention

4.) Using the power of positive thinking to reduce pain and help with the emotional struggles of living with arthritis.

The natural treatments I've included in this book are the ones that I have personally found to be life changing and I hope you will too! *Remember: your life does not have to be limited or hindered just because you have arthritis. The methods in this book can have dramatic effects on your inflammation, mobility, and quality of life!*

Understanding Arthritis

No matter what battle you're fighting, it's important to know the nature of the beast! This short section is designed to help you understand your condition so you know what you're dealing with before you take action – do not worry, I am keeping this section very brief and to the point, this is not never ending medical jargon!

Arthritis is a condition that causes swelling and inflammation in the joints. It can affect any joint in the body and may also cause pain in the muscles, connective tissue, tendons, and ligaments surrounding the joints. Contrary to popular belief, arthritis is not limited to individuals in their senior years. There are a large variety of types of arthritis which can affect people of any age, race, or gender. Approximately 1 in 5 people are diagnosed with some form of arthritis; one third of whom have developed limitations to their work ability. Approximately one third of arthritis sufferers struggle with anxiety and depression. They may have a limited ability to do every day actives; things as simple as walking, bending, and even standing still! Living with arthritis can cause serious financial strain due to medical costs and loss of wages in people who have become unable to work.

As there are so many different types of arthritis, in this book I will talk specifically about *rheumatoid arthritis* **(RA)** and *osteoarthritis* **(OA)**; however, the treatments in this book are relevant to many other arthritic and inflammatory conditions including fibromyalgia, psoriatic arthritis, repetitive strain injuries, and a number of autoimmune conditions that affect the joints and connective tissue.

Osteoarthritis (OA) is a condition of the joints caused by injury, repetitive strain, and years of breakdown of the fluid and cartilage in the affected joint. This type of arthritis will usually affect one or more specific joints. It most often affects the joints in the hands, hips, knees, and spine. Because of its connection with past injury and/or the overworking of a joint, OA rarely affects both sides of the body. The pain associated with osteoarthritis can range from mild to debilitating. It may become worse with activity or may cause a constant ache.

Rheumatoid Arthritis (RA) is a condition which can affect any joint at any time of life. It is caused by an autoimmune process wherein the immune system confuses the body's healthy tissue with harmful substances and attacks them. As the illness progresses, the overactive immune system eventually breaks down the joints causing permanent damage to them. People with RA may suffer from other autoimmune conditions simultaneously. The pain associated with RA most usually affects both sides of the body such as both hands, shoulders, hips, knees, or feet. It can cause constant soreness, stiffness, and fatigue, or it may come and go. Most people living with RA will experience periodic flare ups that can range from mild to severe and may cause every joint in the body to become sore and stiff simultaneously.

A very important part of treating arthritis is taking into account how much it varies from person to person. Although there are many similarities among arthritis sufferers, most people will have a slightly different experience than others. You may have certain joints that are worse than others, you will have different flare up triggers, your pain may be only slightly disruptive or it may cause extremely limited mobility. Most importantly, your life is different from other people's lives. This means everything from your support system, the climate you live in, the type of arthritis you have, your age, what sort of lifestyle you have, and endless other qualities specific to you.

Some common effects of arthritis include:
* Stiff and swollen joints
* Limited mobility
* Limited dexterity
* Mild to severe pain which may worsen with rest, exercise, climate, and other factors
* Insomnia
* Fatigue
* Feelings of heaviness in the body
* Inability to work or travel
* Loss of enjoyment in life
* Depression
* Low motivation
* Frustration and embarrassment

As I'm sure you know, living with arthritis is not easy! Its unpredictable nature can cause serious disruption to your daily life. Daily pain, stiffness, and flare-ups can make it difficult or impossible for you to work, travel, or even accomplish simple household tasks. With close to 40% of people suffering with RA giving up employment because of their condition, you can imagine the added stress and frustration this illness can cause. This could mean not only suffering the discomfort and anxieties of the condition, but also having to face financial concerns and the possibility of giving up one's career or passion. RA sufferers include people of all ages and backgrounds. Your condition may be causing you to steer clear of making plans because you don't know how you'll feel on any given day. You might feel like your life revolves around being ill and this can cause periods of low mood, hopelessness, and anxiety.

Why It's Important To Do What You Can

The fact is, there is no *complete* cure for arthritis but that's no reason to be complacent! There are many, many things you can do - outside of just taking your medication - that can reduce pain and inflammation, slow down the progression of your condition, and even put it into remission. (I know, it happened to me!) At the very least, there are a ton of practical things you can do to simply make your condition easier to live with.

I will never suggest that you go against your doctor's advice and you should always consult your physician before implementing any major changes to your diet or lifestyle. It's important to remember that each of us is different. You know your body best. If you have another condition such as diabetes or high blood pressure that may be exacerbated by a new diet and/or exercise regimen, always seek medical advice before taking action.

Whether you've suffered from arthritis for many years or you've just been diagnosed, there are many things you can do to make a difference. You have more power over your condition than you think! Although the medication and painkillers your doctor gives you may help to reduce your pain and stiffness significantly, you don't have stop there! Arthritis and other inflammatory conditions respond well to a large range of natural treatments. By doing a little bit of work on your end, you might double the effectiveness of the regime your doctor has you on. I promise you, there is hope!

People rarely realize that arthritis is something that you can both improve and slow down. It tends to be thought of as something you simply *have*; like the color of your eyes or your shoe size. Believing that there's nothing you can do about your condition apart from taking your medicine and hoping for the best can really make you feel helpless, hopeless, frustrated, embarrassed, and limited; especially during flare ups or when you realize you can no longer do something you love. It can make you feel like you have no control over your life and that things will never be the same again. It can cause depression and anxiety and put added strain on your family and other close relationships. Living with arthritis can make you feel like you have to give up certain hopes and dreams. It can make you worry about your children or other family members who rely on you. But all is not lost, do not give up hope!

Being involved with your treatment is a great way to gain some power and control over your arthritis. Taking an active part in your treatment means grabbing hold of the reins and saying, **"I deserve better than this."** When you decide to do something about your condition, you're fighting back! You're sending a positive message to yourself and challenging unhelpful negative thoughts. Having some control over your illness is empowering! It can bring a sense of peace and hope back into your life.

Solving The Curse Of Flare Ups

Despite the fact that arthritis is a chronic condition, for most people, it tends to come and go to some extent. You may find that your pain levels change regularly or that you have good days and bad days. Most people living with arthritis experience periodic flare ups during which their pain levels become severe or debilitating. These times can be very unpredictable and may cause major disruptions to your life as well as your mood. Flare-ups can last anywhere from one day to many weeks but they are almost always temporary. Depending on what type of arthritis you have, your flare-ups may affect one or more specific joints or every joint at once. For people living with RA, a flare up can feel like having a bad case of the flu in your entire body.

There are a number of triggers that could kick your condition into high gear. These triggers vary from person to person but generally range from things that are out of your control such as air pollution and the weather to self-imposed things like one's dietary habits, alcohol and caffeine consumption, smoking, and other lifestyle factors. It's not always easy to figure out what factors are contributing to your flare-ups. They may seem to come from nowhere! However, identifying some potential triggers to your condition is a key point to learning how to control it.

Flare-ups can be discouraging and disruptive. They may come regularly or rarely. When you're in the middle of a flare up you can start to feel discouraged and even scared that your condition is worsening. You might be concerned about how to best take care of yourself so as to avoid injury or further illness. You might feel that you have done something wrong to cause your flare up or you may fear that you'll never get better. It can be very hard to see beyond your condition when things are bad.

Although flare-ups can cause worry, pain, and fatigue, it's important that you get plenty of rest until things ease up. Remind yourself that your flare up will eventually cease and that things will settle down again. More than anything though, you can make a big difference to your flare-ups by finding out what underlying triggers are behind them. Understanding your triggers will help you manage your condition better. Being able to recognize what external forces are at work is the first step in discovering how to eliminate them. Later, you will find a large section in this book dedicated to discovering and eliminating triggers, but for now, try the following diary-keeping exercise to start learning what things could be triggering your flare ups.

Know Your Triggers – The First Step To Escaping The Pain

You can get to know what things may be causing your flare-ups by keeping a diary. Do not fret, I will not be asking you to do endless written lists, but it is **vital** to recognize your triggers. Over a course of three to four weeks keep a log of the following things each day:

* What you eat
* How much alcohol you consume
* How much caffeine you consume
* The weather
* Your quality of sleep
* How much you rest your affected joint(s)
* How much you exercise your affected joint(s)
* Any illnesses such as colds, flus, or other infections
* Any stomach upsets

Each morning, afternoon, and evening rate your pain levels from 1-10. Make notes of any significant changes in your energy levels or your mood. Make additional notes of any other bodily discomforts such as headaches or disruptions in your digestive tract.

Once you've kept your diary for a few days or weeks, look for any patterns that suggest a connection between increases and decreases in your pain levels. Ask yourself the following questions:

* Do your pain levels consistently rise after eating certain foods or changes in the weather? * Do they drop when you've been more active or after you've rested?
* Do your pain levels change often or do they remain the same most of the time?

If you see a direct correlation between an external force and an increase to your pain, that may be a trigger to avoid. Similarly, if you find that something is having a positive effect on your condition, increase your exposure to that thing. Continue to write down the effects of your revised lifestyle in your diary.

This exercise is a very basic, stripped down version of the methods this book follows. Doing this initial exercise may not make a massive difference to your pain levels but it's a great way to get into the habits of listening to your body, thinking actively about what is aggravating it, and responding to its needs. As I mentioned earlier, arthritis varies person to person and this is mostly because people's lives and triggers vary person to person! The things that cause you pain (and similarly, those which offer you pain relief) will in many ways reflect your lifestyle and the severity of your condition. This short exercise is an important part of your journey to wellness. Keeping a diary provides you with a tool that will help you gauge changes in your condition as you experiment with changes to your diet and other daily routines. A lot of this book focuses on what you're eating and what your daily activities are. If you try to remember what you had for breakfast, lunch, and dinner last Monday, chances are, you've forgotten by now! Keeping a diary simply makes it easier to keep track of what you're doing so you can identify both your triggers, as well as those things that offer you pain relief; thus making you able to treat your condition faster and more efficiently so you can get on with your life!

After you've done this first exercise, be sure to keep your diary in a safe so that you can look back over it as time goes on. If possible, continue to write in your diary while making changes to your daily routines so that you continue to get a realistic view of what things are helping or harming you. If you are having a flare up, look back over your diary and make a note of what things may have contributed to it. Look for any subtle changes to your wellbeing that may have been signs of an oncoming flare up. Eventually, when you are able to sense the start of your flare-ups, you might be able to stop them before they escalate.

Remember that, although keeping a diary can be tedious, it's important to stick with it. Your condition is specific to you and that means that your diary will be one of the most helpful books you ever read! Managing your arthritis through natural means will take some time before you start feeling a difference. It will take longer than swallowing a pain pill, but I promise, the effects will last longer!

Eventually, with dedication to your new lifestyle, you should find that your flare-ups are less frequent and less severe.

The Tiny Changes That Make A Huge Difference!

Before I go on to the more intricate methods that eventually put my condition into remission, I want to offer you some practical support and subtle changes that can make a substantial difference to your condition and your quality of life. Most of the tips and tricks in this section can be implemented into anyone's daily life quite easily. Some are more complex than others and may involve a little bit of planning and dedication but overall, the important thing is that you do what's right for you! One thing that I will focus on a lot throughout this section and later in this book is maintaining a positive mental attitude. Arthritis can get you down and sometimes just treating your body isn't enough. Taking care of your emotional wellbeing is equally as important as managing your pain.

In this section I've laid out advice in a few lists so that you can refer easily back to these pages when you need to refresh your memory. This way, rather than taking up all your time with basics, you can learn these simple ideas easily and get on to the more substantial stuff quickly. This first list covers fifteen easy things you can do to make a difference to your pain levels every day no matter who you are.

15 Simple Ways To Start Healing Today!

1.) Move more
The pain caused by arthritis might make you want to avoid the use of your stiff and sore joints; however, not using your joints can cause them to stiffen up more and may cause them and their surrounding muscles to degenerate. This can lead to an increase in pain and a decrease in strength and mobility meaning you may become unable to open jars, tie your shoes, walk, or drive a car. Movement is a very

important part of treating arthritis and often the hardest one to get used to. You can maintain your mobility by keeping active and continuing to use your affected joints as much as possible. This may be difficult at the start, especially if you've been avoiding the use of certain joints, but moving is an important start to regaining and maintaining your mobility. Think of it this way: *Move it, or Lose it!*

2.) Manage your weight
If you are overweight, your weight bearing joints such as your hips, knees, and ankles will suffer as a result. You can make a significant difference to your joint pain by maintaining a healthy weight through diet and exercise. If you are unsure how to safely lose weight, ask your doctor or consult a dietitian for advice. Weight management plays a vital role in treating your condition naturally. Taking the weight off your joints could reduce your pain significantly while simultaneously helping with other weight related illnesses. Keeping your weight under control is a vital part of treating your arthritis and your overall wellbeing.

3.) Get plenty of sleep
Approximately two thirds of people suffering with arthritis also suffer from insomnia or other sleep disturbances. This is often due to pain and discomfort and can therefore be difficult to overcome. Unfortunately, getting a poor quality or low quantity of sleep can cause increased pain, mood disruption, and even accelerate joint damage. Do what you can to ensure you're getting enough sleep. Make sure that your mattress is comfortable by purchasing a memory foam mattress or mattress-topper. Use pillows that offer proper neck and shoulder support. Try drinking a herbal tea such as valerian root tea before bed to help your body relax. Keep your bed warm by using an electric blanket or hot water bottle and keep your bed free from obstructions. Try to stay on a regular schedule of sleeping and waking so that your natural body clock kicks in and makes sleeping easier.

4.) Eat well
A diet full of processed or poor quality foods will have a negative effect on your overall wellness. This could mean dramatically increased inflammation and difficulty recovering from flare-ups.

Give your body the right fuel to fight your condition by eating a balanced diet with plenty of fruits and vegetables and as little processed and junk foods as possible. Later in this book I will discuss diet at length so you can be sure you're giving your body all it requires but for now, try to get rid of the junk and increase the greenery!

5.) Keep hydrated
Water is vital to the health all your body systems as it helps nutrients move through your blood
into your joints and organs. It also helps flush toxins out of your system, keeping your joints and organs clear of waste products. You should be drinking at least six to eight glasses of water a day in order to keep your body in top condition. Reduce your intake of sugary drinks, black tea, coffee, and alcohol and *always treat your thirst with water first.*

6.) Take supplements
There are a number of herbal supplements and vitamins that can help with joint pain and inflammation including glucosamine, magnesium, omega 3 fatty acids, and vitamin D. Later in this book I will cover these in detail but you can begin by taking a good quality multivitamin and making sure you're diet includes plenty of variety in vitamin rich fruits and vegetables.

7.) Stay safe
Avoid overusing your joints by recognizing when a task is unsafe for you. If your joints feel weak or sore, ask for help when it comes to lifting heavy objects or doing any other activity that puts too much strain on you. You can also stay safe by using your body weight to open doors rather than relying on your wrists or arms. Use a step stool to reach things that are out of reach rather than stretching awkwardly in ways that may cause you pain. Always bend at the knees when retrieving something from the ground rather than risking back pain. When lifting, hold heavy objects close to your body to reduce strain on your spine. When dressing yourself, sit on a chair for extra stability.

8.) Just say 'No'

Prioritize the tasks you must accomplish each day and don't put too much pressure on yourself to accomplish more than you realistically can. Expending too much energy on things that may hurt you will only exacerbate your inflammation and may cause you increased frustration. Divvy your energy out throughout the day rather than doing too much too fast. Say 'no' to tasks that are too challenging for you and ask for help where needed.

9.) Modify your home
Change your house in ways that will make life easier and safer. Keep things you use often at a level that you can reach without stretching or bending. Keep your floors free of trips and fall hazards. Create larger walkways throughout your home to avoid bumps and bruises. If you struggle considerably with your mobility, consider modifying your home so that you will not need to climb stairs. Install a shower seat and hand railings where there are stairs or inclines.

10.) Get logistical support
Get some help around the house by hiring someone to help with cleaning duties and gardening. Ask friends or family members to help you with things you find particularly difficult to avoid injury or added pressure on sore joints. Getting help will not only make things easier physically; it will also alleviate some of the anxiety and frustration that comes with physical struggles.

11.) Get emotional support
Living with arthritis can have negative effects on your mood and your outlook on life. It's important to have someone you can talk to about your daily struggles so as not to get buried beneath frustration and sadness. Consider talking to a therapist or joining a support group for people living with similar conditions. Often, just taking the time to simply talk to someone else can make a big difference to your mood. A support group could also help you learn some practical ways to make things easier too. If you're not keen on talking to strangers, confide in a close friend, partner, or family member about your feelings.

12.) Keep warm

Most people with arthritis find that staying warm is a necessary component to keeping inflammation at bay. There are a number of ways you can keep your joints warm and loose including wearing multiple layers of clothing in cold weather, wearing gloves in or out of the house, wearing thick socks, sitting by a fire or radiator, taking a hot bath, hugging a hot water bottle, or simply making the most out of a warm day by sitting outside in the sun.

13.) Meditate
Meditation and other stress-reducing activities such as tai chi, yoga, and Pilates can dramatically help with pain, anxiety, low mood, and sleep disturbances. There are many ways you can become involved with mediation including joining a local meditation group, attending guided meditation classes, and listening to relaxation CDs at home. Taking the time to meditate and relax is a great way to maintain a positive mental attitude and this can have a dramatic effect on your physical wellbeing.

14.) Wear insoles or support braces
If you experience chronic pain in your hips, knees, or feet, you may benefit from purchasing insoles or shoes with a thick, flexible sole to help absorb impact when you're walking. A sore wrist, ankle, elbow, or knee may require the help of a support brace during flare-ups. Use ice or heat packs directly on sore joints for extra pain relief. Wearing support braces all the time is not recommended as it can cause the muscles to become weaker so make sure you're only wearing them when you really need to. Many people who suffer from chronic wrist pain find that wearing support braces overnight is enough to reduce daily pain considerably.

15.) Get a massage or acupuncture
Acupuncture and massage can work wonders on sore joints and muscles. In addition to relieving pain, both of these natural techniques also release tension and encourage relaxation which means increased mobility, better moods, and better quality of sleep. Massage and acupuncture are also beneficial for migraines, fatigue, and stress management. The use of a **Transcutaneous Electrical Nerve Stimulation (TENS)** machine may used in conjunction with

either of these practices to help block pain messages being sent to the brain and encouraging the production of endorphins.

Rest vs. Exercise: The Fine Balancing Act!

When your arthritis is flaring up or if your joints seem to hurt constantly, it's natural to want to rest your affected joints. Many people living with chronic pain spend the majority of their lives in bed because they find moving difficult and painful. However, resting your joints too much is not always the best solution. In fact, spending too much time resting could increase your stiffness and pain and may even be one of the causes behind it. Most forms of arthritis and other inflammatory conditions like fibromyalgia respond very favorably to movement. Joints which are in a constant state of stiffness need regular "loosening up" to keep them from seizing. Even people suffering from OA and another forms of arthritis caused by injury or repetitive strain, could benefit greatly from an increase in movement. It's important to learn to recognize when you're resting too much and begin to coerce those sore and stiff joints back into action.

This is not to suggest that you should attempt to run a marathon, nor am I suggesting that becoming mobile again will be easy! If you've spent years of your life not moving, it will take some time to get your body back into action. Like anything new, starting to move over-rested joints will take time and gentle persuasion.

Remember: everyone's condition is unique to them. You may be reading this book as someone who has been living with arthritis for decades or you may still be at the very beginning. Everyone's pain and triggers are different, and everyone's lifestyles are specific to them. Recognizing whether you're resting too much isn't exactly black and white. For some, resting too much could mean spending weeks lying in bed, for others it might be something far more subtle, like avoiding the use of an affected wrist or simply walking less.

And just to make things even more complicated, over-resting isn't the only danger you have. It's also possible to aggravate your arthritis by over-using your joints! When I look back over my first decade living with RA, I can see that I was guilty of both over-resting *and* over-using my joints. I was in my twenties and although I was definitely experiencing pain and limited mobility, I was also not accepting my condition emotionally. I didn't want to believe that anything was "really" wrong with me. This meant that I swung wildly between periods of abundant rest and extreme exercise. At times, I spent weeks in bed wallowing in pain and sadness. Then when things loosened up, I would deny the fact that anything was "wrong" with me at all. I exercised like a fiend, worked long hours, went out and socialized, drank too much, and generally carried on as if I would never feel pain again.

Needless to say, neither of these extreme behaviors did me any good. By the time I entered my thirties, my condition had progressed substantially. My flare-ups were lasting longer and I didn't seem to ever fully recover from them. Although my denial still reared its ugly head at times and sent me back into patterns of over-using my joints, for the most part it was over-resting that took over. I cancelled my gym membership and avoided all forms of structured exercise. I didn't lift, twist, or bend at all because I often suffered with back pain and didn't want to aggravate it or hurt myself. Then I started taking the bus to work rather than walking. Soon I stopped socializing, and eventually I found myself pretty isolated. The fact is, looking back I can see that the less I moved, the less I was *able* move. I gained weight and that caused even more pain in my hips and knees. As my core muscles became weaker and weaker, my back pain also increased. My general health was also at an all time low. I was constantly fatigued and always seemed to be fighting some sort of illness.

Eventually I realized that I needed to get realistic about my condition. I definitely needed to spend less time in bed but I couldn't figure out how that was even possible with my pain levels being so high. I was scared that if I did too much I'd send myself into a flare up but at the same time I knew that I was resting way too much.

Treating your arthritis naturally requires a pretty tricky balancing act where rest and exercise are concerned!

It's important for you to consider, honestly, if you might be resting too much, exercising too much, or doing a little bit of both. Ask yourself the following questions:

1.) Do you rest for long periods of time without getting up to stretch or move?
2.) Are you spending days on end avoiding movement?
3.) Do you avoid the use of a certain joint or joints?
4.) Do you feel that you are getting enough exercise?
5.) Do you fill your "good days" with more physical activity than necessary?
6.) Do you work a physical job or have a physically demanding home life?
7.) Do you take time to rest and recover after periods of heavy activity?
8.) Do you think you're exercising more than you should?

Remember to be completely honest with yourself when assessing your current behaviors. Recognizing if you're resting or exercising too much is paramount to making a change to both your pain levels and your mobility. After taking some time to assess your habits of rest and exercise, consult the following two lists to help you make some subtle changes that could have huge and lasting effects on your stiff and sore body. Read both lists to ensure that you're achieving the best possible balance for you. Remember that "rest" doesn't just mean time spent in bed. It refers to any time you spend not using your affected joints including time spent wearing support straps or braces. "Over-using" your affected joints might include times you continue doing something that you know is causing you pain as well as putting unrealistic pressure on yourself when your body needs to take it easy.

A Healthy Rest / Exercise Balance Is Achievable

For Over-Rested Joints:

1.) Keep warm
One of the reasons resting your joints can increase your pain levels is because joints and muscles stiffen and tighten when they are cold. Just like you would do before an exercise classes, "warming up" your joints and muscles before starting to move them will help loosen them up and reduce the risk of injury. Keep yourself warm with blankets, hot water bottles, and portable heaters; however, don't stop there! Some gentle movement will help warm your joints from the inside out. If you are lying in bed, try to move your affected joints regularly while you're nice and warm. Stretch your arms and legs. Rotate your wrists and ankles. Bend your knees and elbows. Do some gentle neck and back stretches.

Before getting up and moving each day - or before doing any strenuous exercise - try warming your joints up with heat pads. You should notice that you need less time to loosen any tension or stiffness this way.

2.) Move regularly
Joints that are allowed to rest too much become increasingly stiff and sore. If you are taking time to rest during a flare up, make sure that you aren't stopping *all* activity. If your whole body is affected, get up every 30-60 minutes for a short walk around the house to loosen up your stiff joints. If just a few specific joints are affected, make sure those joints get some movement throughout the day. This doesn't mean you should hurt yourself or try to do too much! Simply allow for some light stretching of your sore joints periodically to prevent them from becoming more painful and stiff. If you are wearing a support brace, take it off periodically and do some gentle stretches for your joint and the surrounding muscles, tendons, and ligaments.

Note: Always listen to your doctor! If you have a serious injury and/or your doctor has told you to keep your support brace on, always do as they have suggested.

3.) Challenge yourself

Often times when arthritis pain flares up it can cause you to go into hibernation. Though your body definitely needs rest during these times, spending too much time lying in bed could cause your mood to plummet. Wellness of the mind is a key ingredient to wellness of the body. For this reason, try to keep your mood up by resisting the temptation to sleep all day or do nothing. Invite friends or family to come spend time with you to keep your thoughts from dipping into frustration or hopelessness. If there are things you can accomplish while you're resting such as responding to emails or paying bills, challenge yourself to do them. If there are small physical tasks that you can do around the house, encourage yourself to get up periodically and tackle them. This might just mean taking a walk to the mailbox or doing a few dishes but the movement will help loosen your stiff joints and the activity will help keep your mind from becoming idle and your mood from dropping. So too, proving to yourself that you can do certain tasks despite your condition will help soothe any frustrations you may feel during hard times.

4.) Do some enjoyable light exercise
If your pain levels aren't too high or you recognize that you're spending a bit too much time resting, make a point to do a little light exercise. This can include things like walking, swimming, stretching, gardening, or using your hands to do arts and crafts. Choose something you enjoy and just make sure to take things nice and easy. Invite a friend or relative along to keep your exercise more fun and less tedious! Remind yourself that movement is an important part of your overall mind / body wellness. Don't let long periods of time pass without exercising. Later in this book, I will discuss exercise at length. For now though, try to get at least *30 minutes of exercise* per day.

5.) Dip into some warm water
Having a nice warm bath or sitting in a hot tub can work wonders on sore joints and muscles. Not only does the warmth help ease your pain and loosen joint stiffness, but water also takes a lot of weight off you making it easier for you move without injuring yourself. Take advantage of all the benefits of a warm bath or hot tub by doing some stretches while you're in there. Rotate your wrists and ankles, roll your shoulders backwards and forwards, bend your knees and

elbows a few times and if you're in a deep enough pool, dip your body slowly up and down to increase movement in your hips and spine.

6.) Use your affected joints

If you have just one or a few specific arthritic joints, you may have gotten into the habit of not using them. For instance, if one of your shoulders is regularly stiff and sore, you may be letting your other one do all the work. If one knee is affected, you may have become accustomed to walking with a limp or using your good knee to climb stairs with. Unfortunately, shifting all the strain onto your better joints may cause them damage or injury. Furthermore, if you continue not using your affected joints and muscles, they will become weaker as time goes by meaning increased stiffness and slower healing times.

Challenge yourself to use your affected joints regularly to keep them supple. For sore hips and lower back pain try to walk without limping as much as possible to retain good alignment of the spine. Go slowly at first and always choose terrain that is straight and even. One of the best ways to eliminate a limp that you've developed out of habit, is by simply picking up the pace a little bit. Remember, it's important to make changes like these *gradually*. The aim is to heal your joints, not to make them more painful! Always slow down or stop when your pain levels rise significantly.

For Over-Worked Joints:

1.) Assess the importance of the task at hand

If you have a ton of things to do, take a minute to prioritize your to-do list. Take some pressure off yourself by lightening your load a bit. Look at the things you have to do and ask yourself how important each task is. If there are things that can wait until tomorrow or next week, give yourself permission to let them go until you're able to do them. This might mean letting the dishes sit in the sink overnight or leaving the grocery shopping until later in the week. If you're prone to doing too much, ask yourself periodically if the task at hand is worth a flare up. If it isn't, it can wait.

2.) Take regular breaks

Whether your pain is in one joint or all of your joints, you will need to let them rest during flare-ups. If you are reluctant or unable to take time off work or other tasks, remind yourself to take breaks regularly. If your whole body is affected, time aside every so often to sit or lay down for 15-30 minutes. If you have a few specific joints that hurt, at least rest those that are affected by using a support brace or treating them with heat or ice. If your schedule is demanding, make a conscious effort to schedule in some rest after work. Treat yourself to a professional massage, a hot bath, or an early bedtime. Make yourself and your joints a priority!

3.) Slow down

If you're the type of person who tries to get everything done as quickly as possible, or your life is particularly demanding, you may be adding unnecessary strain to your joints by trying to get too much done at once. It's important to let yourself slow down when your pain is flaring up. Remind yourself that if you continue moving at your normal pace, your flare up could last longer than necessary. Similarly, do not pressure yourself into doing the same amount of work when your joints are particularly bad. Whether it's work, family life, the gym, or social obligations, putting too much pressure on yourself with only increase your pain and lengthen your flare-ups. Slow things down to give your body the rest it needs.

4.) Manage your tasks

If your to-do list is unavoidable, schedule your tasks around your pain. If your pain is flaring up, assess the jobs you have to do and take care of the things on your list won't hurt you such as emailing, admin, and organization. Leave the physical work until you're feeling better. If your pain is particularly bad in the morning, let yourself rest and move slowly until you're more mobile. Then get on to the harder jobs on your list.

5.) Get help

Having too much to do during a flare up could put a lot of pressure on you. It may cause you stress and frustration that may lead to low mood and/or physical exhaustion. If there are things you need to do but your arthritis is making them difficult, ask someone for help. This can be hard for people who are used to doing things on their own but your joints will thank you for it! Try to discuss your condition with family and friends so that they can better understand how to help you when you're having a hard time. Try to delegate tasks that other people can handle both at work and at home so as to ensure you're in good enough condition to take care of the things that really matter. Consider having your groceries delivered or using a cleaning service to help with things around the house. Getting help doesn't need to hurt your pride. *You should feel proud about making yourself a priority!*

6.) Listen to your body
Make regular assessments of your pain from 1-10. If something is causing you pain above a level 5, either take a break until you're feeling better, ask someone else to help you with it, or slow down to let your joints do the work more easily. It's very important for you to get to know your condition. That includes triggers and unhelpful habits, but it also includes recognizing when you're doing something right! If you find relief from one of the treatments in this book, stick with it! Similarly, if you try something and find that it's not making a difference for you, try something else. Listening to your body and recognizing its signals is of upmost importance when it comes to managing your symptoms.

Being Good To Your Body

When treating your arthritis naturally, it's important to look at the big picture. Unfortunately, arthritis isn't like a splinter. It can't simply be removed and thrown away. Arthritis is more complicated than that. When in remission, sometimes it seems that arthritis is just waiting for a reason to rear its ugly head. During flare-ups, it can knock you down completely. Therefore, treating arthritis naturally takes planning and dedication. Most importantly, if you really want to see the end of your arthritis, you have to look at the bigger picture.

Imagine your condition like a quiet predator. It lurks in the background of your life, you may hear a threatening growl from it now and again, and every once in a while, it strikes. And when it does, it can be devastating; often causing extreme pain, limited mobility, and increased weakness against future attacks. In order to protect yourself from the predator and prevent it from striking, you need a strong defence. By changing the conditions surrounding your arthritis, you can diminish the possibility of it striking! What I'm talking about here is focusing on your full body wellness, because when your body is in its healthiest state, your arthritis is far less likely to knock you down. Getting your body to its optimal health will make your flare ups less intense and less frequent. Your daily aches and pains will also subside.

You may have noticed (especially if you suffer from RA or another autoimmune condition) that one small compromise in the body can lead to lengthy periods of illness. For instance, let's say everyone in your home gets a cold. It's natural for you to also be affected, but chances are, when you get the cold, it's a little more complicated. While your body tries to fight off the infection, your arthritis might take the opportunity to make things more difficult for you. You might experience inflammation in some or all of your joints, you may feel like you have the flu, your body may become heavy and stiff, and you might even experience a full on flare up. You may find that you need to stay in bed for days on end and that your recovery takes longer than the other people in your household. This could also lead to a succession of illness as the body struggles to regain its health. So what can you do to make sure your common cold doesn't progress into something worse? The answer is simple: *Focus on total body wellness every day.*

By treating your whole body constantly - rather than just when your arthritis is flaring up - you are eliminating the possibilities for your arthritis to knock you down. By treating your body right and living a healthy lifestyle, you'll experience longer periods of wellness and your body will be better equipped to fight common illnesses. You'll heal faster from infections and injury, and most importantly, by being good to your body, you could send your arthritis into remission for weeks, years, or even forever.

Most people know that a diet full of fatty and unhealthy foods could be damaging to their health. Yet, the average diet (both in the US, and the UK) is rich in junk foods, fast foods, and processed foods. This means high levels of salt, sugar, simple carbohydrates, and both saturated and trans fats, not to mention a severe lack in vital nutrients, "good" fats, "friendly bacteria", and antioxidants.

Over the last century or so, changes to what we eat and how it's produced has meant that a shocking amount of foods in our grocery stores - despite being approved by the FDA - are simply, not good for you. Our diets have changed dramatically in the last few decades. Today, up to 90% of the food consumers are buying in the United States are lacking in essential nutrients. In addition to eating an abundance of processed foods, nearly 75% of Americans are eating less than five portions of fruit and vegetables a day. It's no wonder conditions like arthritis are more common now than they were just a few generations ago!

The truth is, healthy eating is not just about body image or looking good on the beach! A diet lacking in natural sources of vital nutrients could cause a variety of health problems; most specifically, joint conditions. Recent studies show a direct correlation between certain foods and inflammation. Trans fats, MSG, artificial sweeteners and colors, homogenized fats, and the lengthy range of sugars on the market (fructose, lactose, corn syrup, sucrose, and dextrose) can all promote disease *and* initiate inflammation. The vast majority of store bought pasta sauces, cereals, soups, Chinese or Indian cooking sauces, snack foods (including those "low fat" or "healthy" varieties), and virtually anything else in your cupboards that isn't a whole food, contain ingredients that could be exacerbating your condition. Furthermore, food that is processed, pre-made, or pre-packaged is often made with ingredients that are of low quality and low cost. Using sugar, salt, and "artificial flavorings" is an cheap and easy way for food production companies to get flavor into processed foods; therefore avoiding their need to use good quality produce. Most of us would like to trust that the food in our supermarkets is safe to eat; but unfortunately that's just not the case.

In addition to the connection between certain foods and inflammation, unhealthy foods can also cause a considerable amount of weight gain. Most people know that obesity can cause heart disease, diabetes, and certain cancers; but few people realize the connection between fat and arthritis. The truth of the matter is that being overweight can exacerbate absolutely every type of arthritis and what's more, excess weight can actually *cause* a number of types of arthritis! Approximately one third of obese people will develop some form of arthritis! Adding strain and pressure to weight-bearing joints will eventually cause them harm. Each pound you gain above a healthy weight causes four times the amount of pressure on your hips, knees, and spine. So, if you're 20lbs overweight, you're actually doing 80lbs worth of damage to your weight-bearing joints. No wonder they hurt so bad!

You can easily imagine how osteoarthritis could be caused by weight gain, but unfortunately if it's RA you're suffering from, it's more complicated than that. Fat releases a number of inflammatory chemicals called "cytokines" into the body. Many of these chemicals promote and cause inflammation in a variety of body systems posing a significant threat to people suffering from RA. Cytokines are also thought to be a factor in RA patients suffering from "cachexia" or muscle wastage; a degeneration that affects around two thirds of RA sufferers (most commonly in the hands and thighs). People suffering from muscle wasting may experiences feelings of tired, heavy, or overworked muscles even during periods of rest. Muscle wasting can cause weight fluctuation as well as loss of strength and mobility. Furthermore, as the heart is also a muscle, RA patients suffering from muscle wasting are at heightened risk for heart failure. It's important to note that even during periods of remission and when pain is being successfully managed, muscle wasting can still be occurring. Later, I will discuss further natural treatments for muscle wasting but the most powerful weapon against it by far, is a healthy diet which is low in saturated and trans fats.

Of all the methods and medications I've used for my RA, nothing has made a difference quite as significant as changing my diet has. Before making the decision to try natural treatments, my condition was progressing rapidly. My flare-ups increased in quantity and severity almost overnight. The pain was excruciating and I found myself bed ridden for days on end at least once a month (often more). It had gotten to a point where I was missing work at least one week out of every month. I couldn't make plans to travel or socialize, and started feeling like my life was not my own.

What's worse was that I had two small children at home who I, frankly, just couldn't keep up with. I stopped being able to play with them and couldn't plan fun days out because I never knew if I'd be mobile enough when the day came. Even cooking dinner or just sitting and helping them with homework was challenging. The pain was everywhere. My shoulders, hands, back, legs, and feet. Even my jaw felt tight and stiff. My flare-ups came suddenly and left me useless for unpredictable amounts of time. And the fact that I had only just turned thirty was a constant reminder that something was "wrong" with me. Arthritis was a constant source of frustration and sadness in my life.

It was around this time that I started to identify as being "sick". My illness had bulldozed me and I was flattened by its weight. I believed it had changed me forever and my life was no longer my own. Being "sick" became the most prominent part of my personality. Sometimes I thought it carried more weight than my name. "Hello, my name is rheumatoid arthritis."

As things progressed I began feeling embarrassed by my condition. The more other people knew about it, and the more they pitied me, the more I felt like there was no hope. I became deeply depressed. It all seemed to be happening so fast too. I couldn't help thinking (and saying) "I'm too young for this!". And as my mood spiraled in and out of despair, my dietary habits spiraled out of control. In my hopeless state, I resigned myself to a lifetime of pain and sickness. Naturally, I tried to "soothe" myself with all the wrong things: alcohol, caffeine, sugar, fat, carbs, you name it! I slept too much or not at all. I told myself that drinking alcohol was helping my pain and that I needed caffeine throughout the days because my energy levels were so low. I skipped meals and then filled myself with breads, cakes, and sweets. I told myself that I "deserved" some treats in life since things were so bad.

As you can imagine, my diet and lifestyle at that time was *not* helping my condition. In fact I was becoming more and more fatigued every day. My flare-ups were getting worse and coming more often. My stomach was constantly upset. My joints were always at least a little sore. I was gaining weight and losing sleep. Eventually I quit my job because my condition had gotten the better of me. My confidence dwindled so much that I stopped seeing friends and family. I became more and more isolated as my hope continued to wane.

By this time I had heard a little bit about how certain foods could aggravate autoimmune diseases and other joint conditions. I had read a few success stories online but I wasn't sure if I actually believed any of them. It seemed like a myth to me. If the medication my doctor had prescribed was barely making me feel better, how would a vitamin tablet or changing my diet have any effect? Also, changing my diet would be hard work and I was so tired all the time that I dreaded the thought of having to learn all new recipes and give up the convenience foods that I thought were making things "easier" on me.

But there came a day when I knew it was time to make a change. I was attending an event at my children's school and I hadn't seen my friends or any other school parents for most of the year. During my time of isolation I had gained thirty pounds and began walking with a cane. I hadn't realized quite how incredible my transformation had been until that evening. I hobbled in and took the seat closest to the door. People who had known me just a few of months ago couldn't believe how much things had changed for me. They stared or offered me pitying smile-frowns and looks of concern. As the other parents in the room talked, laughed, and ran after their little ones I was sitting like a hospital patient longing for my bed. It all became very real to me that night. I didn't want this illness. I wanted to be happy and light like other people. I had to be good to my body. I had to fight back.

I started researching ways I could get my condition under control. I didn't think about giving up my medication or magically curing myself, but I was sure there was something else I could do that would make a difference. Doing the research was confusing at times. There seemed to be a number of potentially helpful natural treatments for all types of arthritis and other autoimmune conditions but most of them had inconclusive results or very little research proving their effectiveness. I also knew that I had to learn more about my condition. I have RA, which I knew was an autoimmune disease, but I didn't know exactly what that meant. Did I need to treat my joints or my immune system? Was there actually such a thing as "remission" in RA? If there was actually a possibility of RA sufferers living a normal life, why hadn't my doctors ever said so? How many people in the world were suffering with similar conditions, helplessly watching their lives slip away?

There was only one way of knowing if there was hope for a recovery and that was to just get stuck in. I decided to start small. I thought that the best way to know if something is making a difference is to try one thing at a time and see how things go. After talking to my doctor about my plans, I bought a few different vitamins that I'd read about online and started implementing them into my daily routine. I started by taking glucosamine (known to help joint lubrication and cartilage repair) and omega 3 (a fatty acid that can help moderate inflammation). I have to say that I found it difficult to get myself into a routine and I did forget to take my vitamins here and there. However, a week or so later, I was definitely beginning to notice some difference to my condition. It wasn't a drastic improvement but it felt like my body was starting to loosen up a bit and that was enough to encourage me to stick with it. I was still a little bit skeptical, but I wouldn't be for long.

The next two supplements I tried - magnesium and vitamin D - made a noticeable difference to my pain levels, sleep patterns, *and* my mood. It was the first significant change I'd had and I cannot even describe how much more positive I was beginning to feel after only two weeks. This change also spurred me on to be more diligent with my glucosamine and omega 3's. I don't know if I ever believed I could get my "old life" back, but for the first time in a long time, I felt like there was hope for a brighter future.

Although many people believe that arthritis is hereditary, there is very little evidence supporting this idea. In fact, quite the opposite appears to be true. The majority of types of arthritis have been actually been proven not to be hereditary. There are certain genetic factors involved in autoimmune conditions which suggest that someone who has a close family relation who suffers from RA or another autoimmune condition could have an increased likelihood of developing it. Ultimately though, research suggests that most types of arthritis (including most autoimmune varieties) are caused by other factors such as hormonal changes, environmental toxins, diet and exercise, longterm smoking habits, vitamin deficiencies, and bacterial or viral infections. Following my marked improvement after starting the magnesium, I did further research and I was intrigued by the possibility that a magnesium deficiency might not only be causing the inflammation in my joints, but that it may even be an underlying cause of my body's autoimmune process as a whole.

Magnesium is an essential mineral that most people are deficient in. I was surprised to find that magnesium doesn't only work well as a natural anti-inflammatory; it's actually a major player in a variety of health concerns. A person who is magnesium deficient could be the victim of a world a problems. Not getting enough of it can cause anxiety and depression, migraines, chronic fatigue, brain and heart conditions, obesity, diabetes, kidney stones, asthma, joint conditions, and more. Having a poor diet - or even just a *typical* diet which includes processed foods and sugary drinks - can contribute to magnesium deficiently but there are also a number of other factors at hand. Alcohol, age, illness, digestive problems, calcium supplements, certain medications, and stress can all contribute to a magnesium deficiency, as well as causing an inability for the body to absorb and use it. At this stage in my journey, I was still just at the tip of the iceberg; but I do believe that taking magnesium supplements made a very significant change to both my condition, and my life.

The other vitamin that I found to make the most significant change at this early stage of my journey was vitamin D. A deficiency in vitamin D can cause a variety of problems including disruptions to the immune system and joint damage. If you're not spending a good bit of time in the sun every day it's quite possible that you could be vitamin D deficient and this was definitely true in my case. Spending so much time in bed limited my exposure to the sun, as did my location and enduring the darker seasons. After having my vitamin D levels checked by my doctor, I learned that they were extremely low. I started taking taking supplements and made it a mission to increase my exposure the sun whenever possible. Sometimes this meant as little as simply sitting in my back yard for ten or fifteen minutes a day but it made an undeniable difference. I found that, as my vitamin D levels increased, my mood was much brighter. I was sleeping better and felt generally more calm. My pain levels also dropped.

It was around this time that I began to feel a lot less agitated about my condition to. I still had pain and I was still experiencing flare-ups but they didn't seem quite as bad and I was definitely coping with them better. I was glad that things seemed like they were easing up but I knew that taking supplements wasn't the best way to get everything my body needed. Relying on supplements just isn't as beneficial as getting what your body needs through a healthy diet and I still had some bad habits to kick if I was going to make a real difference. So I conducted more research and got to work!

Before I go on to tell you the next great leap in my recovery, here's a recap of the first few steps I made in taking control of my arthritis and why they worked for me:

1.) I made the decision to be good to my body
Before I began my journey I had given up. I had let my illness define me and I was miserable. Making the decision to be good to my body meant doing a lot of research and being committed to myself and my future. It wasn't easy but I knew that doing *something* was better than doing *nothing*! Although my story is personal and unique to me - as yours will be to you - I believe that anyone who wants to make a difference in their condition must make a commitment to being kind to their body.

2.) I started taking glucosamine supplements

Glucosamine is essential joint repair and cartilage maintenance and it may help slow joint damage as well. People suffering from most forms of arthritis will get some benefit from it. Glucosamine is available in capsules, liquids, and powder form. Most supplements are sourced from shellfish; however there are plant-based alternatives which should be used in the case of a shellfish allergy or strict vegetarian diet.

Note: Glucosamine may increase blood sugar, so if you are diabetic, always seek advice from a doctor before taking it.

3.) I started taking omega 3 supplements
Omega 3 fatty acids are essential for brain health but they have also proven to be excellent for inflammation and pain. Research shows they may also help suppress the immune system as well which means they're particularly helpful for people suffering from RA and other autoimmune conditions. Omega 3's are most commonly found in fish oils but there are also a variety of plant-based sources including as walnuts, seeds, leafy greens, cruciferous vegetables, and squash. Both fish oils and vegetarian omega 3's are available in capsule form as well.

4.) I starting taking magnesium supplements
This is a powerful yet underrated mineral that provides a world of health benefits. Magnesium plays an integral role in calcium absorption but unlike calcium, it does not store itself in the body, meaning it must be replenished daily. There are a number of food sources of magnesium including whole grains such as brown rice, buckwheat, and rye, as well as legumes, nuts, and green vegetables. However, to optimize your magnesium intake, you may want to take a daily supplement in capsule form. Magnesium is also available in an oil which you spray directly on your skin. This is a great option to use in place of an oral supplement as it absorbs easily into the body without putting any excess strain on your digestive tract. I have found that spraying magnesium directly on my sore joints provides relief in seconds!

5.) I increased my exposure to vitamin D

This elusive vitamin is most easily gotten from sun exposure which means that depending on your location and the season, you could be deficient. Studies have shown that that there is a significant link between Vitamin D deficiency and arthritis pain. In fact, the majority of people suffering from autoimmune diseases are vitamin D deficient. In addition to its effect on arthritis, vitamin D is also beneficial for other illnesses including depression, cancer, and heart disease. Vitamin D can be hard to get through diet alone, so in order to maximize levels in your body, increase the amount of time you spend in the sun (taking care to apply sunscreen after a short period of exposure). If your lifestyle or geographical location don't allow for this, consider taking a daily supplement to ensure healthy levels. If in doubt, have your levels tested by a doctor and ask for advice on how much you should take.

Learning How To Eat Right & The Colossal Changes It Can Make

Although taking vitamin supplements did help my condition, I knew that trying to get all the all vitamins and minerals my body needed through supplements wasn't good enough. There was a lot more I could do to improve my condition and it was time to get started. So, back to researching I went!

What I found this time around was even *more* inconclusive theories and conflicting reports! One article would say to avoid a certain food while the next article claimed that food was a miracle cure! The sheer amount of information on the internet really paints a picture of just how many people are affected by these conditions and how hopeless things can seem. The further I read and researched, some things did begin to make sense; it was getting easier to see the difference between the myths and the hard evidence. But there was still quite a lot of conflicting reports found in case studies and this led me to believe that joint pain, arthritis, and autoimmune conditions in general are not exactly straight forward. On the contrary, there seems an unending amount of complexity and variety surrounding these conditions. Despite a few key similarities, it seems that just about everyone has a slightly different experience with arthritis including varying causes, pain levels, mobility, and treatment success which brings me back to stressing why it's important to do what works for *you* and *your* condition. But don't worry. I'm not going to leave you high and dry! Rather, I'm going to show you how I found what worked for me so you can find out what's going to work for you. I want to note here again that although I talk about RA quite a lot in this book, the advice here will also be helpful for those suffering from OA and a variety of other joint conditions.

When it comes to natural treatments you may need to go through a certain amount of trial and error before you know exactly what you're doing and why. I am of the belief system that if something is improving your condition, it's worth sticking with. And conversely, if something you're doing or consuming is contributing to your pain and stiffness, put a stop to it. The problem for most people is knowing where to start, and that's exactly why I've written this book!

Here's how I discovered the culprits behind my inflammation, pain, and fatigue:

Step One: Detox

"Detox" is a word we hear a lot these days and most of us think of it as a quick way to lose weight or recover from a big night out! However, detoxing your system is actually about flushing out harmful waste products that have built up in your body systems (including your joints and connective tissue). Harmful toxins in your diet and your environment can cause and contribute to your pain and inflammation. In fact, taking a quick look at the history of arthritis paints a whole new picture of why we suffer from these illnesses in the first place.

It's interesting to know that there are little to no historical accounts of rheumatoid arthritis in the centuries preceding the industrial age and though there have been a few rare accounts of illnesses similar to arthritis, examinations of medieval skeletons in the UK have turned up no signs of the disease whatsoever. In fact, it wasn't until the mid 1800's that RA was given its name; just under twenty years after the start of the industrial revolution. Theoretically, this suggests that changes to the environment caused by industrial factories could've been a major catalyst for RA along with many other health conditions. It's no great secret that the industrial revolution caused some devastating effects to our environment; many of which are still around today. Factories emitted poisonous substances into the earth, our water sources, and the air we breathe. The clearing of trees for use in factories only exacerbated the problem as it greatly reduced the amount of oxygen and clean air that humans and other species (many of which are now extinct) needed to survive. Studies on many communities around the world have shown a direct correlation between urbanization and arthritis. People living in urban or more "developed" areas of the world are exposed to far more toxins than those living in extreme rural conditions. And it is these people who making up the majority of people suffering from joint problems. Factory emissions, vehicle exhaust, chemical cleaners, exposure to pesticides, mass produced cheap foods, landfills, and hundreds of other things in our daily lives are causing levels of toxins in our environment that can have a detrimental effect on our health.

But it's not just the air we breathe that's putting toxins into our systems. Our diets could be the most significant factor when it comes to toxins and related illnesses. Most of us are aware that eating too much fatty, salty, or sugar foods could have negative effects on your weight and overall health. Unfortunately though, with the pace of the world nowadays, sometimes we're so busy it seems like the only options for dinner are popping a ready meal in the microwave or throwing a jar of tomato sauce over some pasta.

Very few people take the time to read the ingredients of every single food item they buy, but if you go to your kitchen right now and read the ingredients of any processed food in your cupboards, you're highly likely to find quite a few unpleasant things on the list such as sugar, salt, preservatives, artificial colors and sweeteners, "flavor enhancers", gelatine, and so-called "natural flavors". In addition, cooking foods at very high temperatures can actually create toxins in them; including vegetables. With that in mind, think of the toxins you could be ingesting when eating "fast food", fried foods, or bbq'ed foods.

In order to get a clearer view of what's causing your pain and inflammation, it's a good idea to start by flushing the toxins out of your system. Toxins come from the food and drink we consume, pollutants in our environment, high stress levels, and chemicals we come across in our daily lives. For most people, toxins are easy enough for their bodies to fight, but people suffering from inflammatory and/or autoimmune conditions could be weaker against them. This means that rather than our bodies fighting toxins the way other people can, when toxins are present in our bodies, our immune systems kick into high gear and start attacking everything in sight - *including* our own cells. So we need to launch a counter-attack! But before you can really build a defence against the substances that are hurting you, you need to start by getting the toxins out of your system!

There are a lot of cleansing fads going around; many of which are simply too difficult to see all the way through. The lists below focus on the most harmful toxins as well as the most helpful detoxifiers. Do your best to stick to these bare minimum requirements to kick your body into gear and get those nasty toxins out of your joints. If you live with family or friends, ask them to detox with you to make the process easier. Their bodies will benefit too! Begin your detoxification by spending two to four weeks on the following simple cleanse.

Cleanse Your System By Avoiding These Inflammation Triggers

*Alcohol
*Caffeine that comes from coffee and black tea (replace with green tea if necessary)
*Refined sugar and all food products containing it
*Dairy and eggs
*Tobacco
*All meats (excepting occasional fatty fish such as salmon or tuna if necessary)
*Saturated Fats (including meat and dairy fats as well as cooking oils)
*Citrus fruits (excepting lemon and limes)
*White varieties of rice and wheat products

Optimize your Cleanse By Increasing Consumption Of These

*Water - try to drink around 3 liters per day
*Herbal teas or warm water with lemon

*Organic fruits
*Organic green, yellow, and orange vegetables - such as broccoli, spinach, and squash
*Omega 3 fatty acids - namely that which is found vegetables and seeds
*Whole grains - choose brown varieties of rice, pastas, and bread products.

In addition to changes in your diet, you can help your detoxification along by exercising, spending time in a sauna or steam room to help your body sweat toxins out, and by getting plenty of rest and relaxation (the best way to combat toxins caused by stress).

Think of your body as using pain and inflammation as a form of communication. If you experience pain, fatigue, headaches, or nausea after eating certain foods, it's likely that your body is sensitive to them and it's trying to tell you so! The problem is, many of us eat the same foods every day so it's hard to know which foods are contributing to your pain and stiffness and which ones may be helping to fight against it.

After your detoxification, your body should be mostly free of toxins meaning you'll be able to see more clearly, the effect your diet has on your arthritis. Think of it as starting at square one. Now that your system is clean, your body can tell you what's aggravating it and you can hear it more clearly and do something about it!

Step Two: Eliminating Food Triggers

When treating your arthritis naturally, one of the most important things to consider is the possibility of one or more food triggers. Many arthritis sufferers have discovered that certain foods and/or certain families of foods wreak havoc on their systems and there is a decent amount of consistency where these reports are concerned. In my case, I found that there were multiple foods causing my flare-ups as well as contributing to my daily aches and stiffness. Discovering these triggers was the most important part of my journey to wellness as I was able to eliminate them from my diet and change my illness entirely. It was through diet that I eventually put my RA into remission, increased my quality of life, and rebuilt my hopes for the future.

In order to find out what foods may be contributing to your pain and inflammation, you will need to begin by eliminating a number of common dietary triggers. Considerable research has shown that by eliminating certain foods, you may be able to reduce inflammation, stiffness, fatigue, headaches, and stomach upsets, as well as sending rheumatoid arthritis and other autoimmune conditions into remission.

When I first began my research I have to admit I was a bit skeptical of all the claims I read about people "curing" their arthritis through natural means. We mustn't forget that there is no "cure" for arthritis of any kind. That is the simple truth of the matter. I will always have RA. But I can say honestly, that my condition is no longer disruptive to my life and I believe the reports of other arthritis sufferers who have had similar experiences. I made a resolved to do whatever I could to make my life with RA easier. And, although I understand that the illness will never fully go away, I have found that it can stay away for quite some time; possibly even forever.

I have to admit that behind my skepticism at the start, there lurked some reluctance. I was nervous about having to let go of some of my favorite foods. What if my very favorite food was the culprit? Would that mean I could never eat it again? Which foods exactly would I have to eliminate? Could I really live without all those things? What will I eat? Will I have to learn how to cook all new foods?! How much time and energy is this all going to take?

The only way to answer any of these questions was to just wait and see. It couldn't hurt to try! I decided to start with a 30 day trial and I'm so glad I did! Finding out what foods were contributing to my condition became my most powerful weapon against it. It gave me freedom from my pain and brought quality back to my life.

Here's what I did:

For 30 days I eliminated ALL possible triggers including:

1.) Gluten
Gluten is a protein found in many cereal grains; most notably, wheat. Many people suffering from RA and other autoimmune conditions have an intolerance or allergy to gluten that can cause inflammation in the digestive tract as well as the joints. It can also be the culprit behind fatigue and regular bouts of stomach upsets and other digestive issues. Therefore, eliminating gluten from your diet may have very positive effects on your both your condition and your energy levels. Most grocery stores and restaurants offer gluten free varieties of breads, pasta, cakes, and other common foods so eliminating gluten is easier than you think!

Note: For people suffering from osteoarthritis, a gluten free diet is unlikely to help your condition, although, if you suffer from regular stomach discomfort or digestive troubles, you may find that it's worth a try!

2.) Processed, fried, and "fast" foods
Foods like frozen ready meals, French fries, and mass-produced "fast" foods often contain ingredients that could contribute to pain inflammation such as high levels of salts, sugars, and animal fats. In addition, foods which have been fried or grilled at high temperatures may contain advanced glycation end product (AGEs) which can cause inflammation as well as damaging certain bodily proteins. Avoid these foods by cooking your meals at home, eating more raw or steamed vegetables, and packing lunches when you're out for the day to avoid buying unhealthy snacks.

3.) Meat
An increasing amount of research has shown that avoiding all meats (including poultry and fish) can have a significant effect on the pain and inflammation associated with arthritis. Many schools of thinking

on the subject suggest that a vegan, gluten-free diet has the greatest effect on the condition. However, there are other studies that encourage simply avoiding red meat as it is a well known arthritis trigger. For the purpose of the 30 day elimination diet, I would urge you to avoid all meat if at all possible so that you can know if it actually is a trigger for your condition. If you find that avoiding all meat is not possible, try to at least avoid all meats apart from fish as it is thought of as the least harmful meat and it may contain some nutrients that can help with joint conditions.

4.) Dairy

Some research has shown that dairy products can have a serious effect on RA and other chronic joint conditions. This is due mainly to the effect dairy has on the digestive tract as it may cause "leaky gut" syndrome (a topic I will discuss at length in the next section of this book), therefore allowing toxins to "leak" into your bloodstream. This can result in fatigue, constant stomach pain, and regular bouts of joint inflammation. Removing dairy from your diet for a short time should help you to notice if it's contributing to your condition. There are a number of vegan alternatives to milk and other dairy products including cheese, yoghurt, and ice cream. As such a great number of people experience intolerances to dairy, it is worth avoiding it during your 30 day elimination diet to clarify whether or not it's affecting you.

Note: For sufferers of osteoarthritis, reducing dairy intake may have little to no effect on your condition. In fact, dairy is generally considered good for joints suffering from degeneration. If you have OA and want to give up dairy, talk to your doctor before making any major changes to your diet.

Nightshades: The Astounding Difference This Can Make

"Nightshade vegetables" are a food group containing a substance called alkaloids which may cause pain, stiffness, poor healing, stomach upsets, insomnia, and arthritis itself. Studies show that

nightshade vegetables are implicated in both RA and OA as well as other inflammatory conditions. The list of nightshades is lengthy and may include some of the most difficult foods to give up; however, in my and many other people's experience, taking nightshades out of your diet can have a dramatic effect on your condition and your daily health.

In my personal journey, I discovered that nightshades were the most offensive foods when it came to my joint pain. Living on a diet which is free of nightshades is not easy but in my experience it is well worth it. The good news is that certain nightshades can prove more offensive than others and there are many arthritis sufferers who are only sensitive to one or two foods in the family. Everyone is different. For instance, I flare up after eating most nightshades but I have found that I can tolerate moderate amounts of blueberries while I'm severely intolerant to potatoes.

The 30 day elimination diet is difficult where nightshades are concerned as they include some of our most common foods; however, I urge you to give it a try.

Nightshades include:
*Tobacco
*Potatoes (all varieties *excluding* sweet potatoes and yams)
*Tomatoes (all varieties)
*Peppers (including all varieties of sweet, bell, hot, cayenne, and paprika; not to be confused with peppercorns which are not nightshades!)
*Eggplant (Aubergine)
*Okra
*Gooseberries
*Goji berries
*Blueberries
*Huckleberries

Reading the list above probably made you ask "how are any of these foods even related?!" and although it may seem like a strange list, all of these foods are members of the family *Solanacea*. A good way to recognize nightshades is by how they grow. Most of them feature a spiky little green "hat" from where they were attached to their plant.

At some point in your life, you may have heard of *"deadly nightshade"*; a rather poetic name for the poisonous *belladonna*. There are quite a few non-edible nightshades in existence which may be considered "deadly", but it does appear that even in the edible nightshades, the same poison lurks in very small doses and acts sort of like a natural "pesticide" to keep the plant away from harm.

Although there is no evidence proving that edible nightshades are *poisonous*, there have been quite a lot of studies which suggest that they can be responsible for joint pain, inflammation, and autoimmune processes. There are a few different theories as to why the correlation exists between arthritis and nightshades ranging from individual intolerances to antagonistic chemicals found in the nightshades themselves. One idea that I feel is significant to the argument is the presence of "leaky gut" and other digestive problems among people living with autoimmune diseases. It appears that the alkaloids contained in nightshades don't just cause stomach upsets. Rather, it is thought that - through "leaky gut" syndrome - the alkaloids may "leak" into the bloodstream and cause an increased immune response. For a person suffering with RA or other conditions where the immune system attacks healthy cells, this could mean adding fuel to an already blazing fire.

The good news is that you can find out if nightshades are causing you problems fairly easily during your 30 day elimination diet. Once you have successfully eliminated possible triggers, you can begin reintroducing them into your system to see how they affect you. If you come to find that you have no problem with some or even all nightshades, you will be able to eat them freely without any ill effect. There is no need to "cut down" or avoid nightshades unless you know they're affecting you badly. Furthermore, very few people find that *all* nightshades have the same effect on them. Most people find that some nightshades make them feel worse than others. Once you've excluded nightshades for a few weeks, you can then experiment with adding them back into your diet one at a time to see which ones, if any, are aggravating your joints.

After reading the list of nightshades, I'm sure you can see why avoiding them can be so difficult! I can tell you from experience that learning to live (and cook) without nightshades can take a lot of getting used to. Not only are nightshades the most commonly eaten produce in most people's diets, but they're also used in the production of most processed foods, often disguised with ambiguous wording like "flavorings", "starch", and "vegetable protein". This can make it impossible to know what's exactly in there! In addition, you will find that quite a lot of every-day foods include tomatoes, peppers, and paprika such as baked beans, soups, ketchup, and BBQ sauce. Potato starch is also found in a number of products such as gluten-free breads, cakes, certain medications, and food supplements. However, living without nightshades is by no means impossible. It simply involves learning some new recipes and developing new habits. If nightshades are affecting you badly, you will probably need to cook more at home rather than eating in restaurants a lot. You may also find it necessary to pack lunches or snacks if you're going out for the day too. The other thing that helps is, the more you listen to your body, the more you'll know how a certain food will affect you. If you're only going to have a slight reaction to a food, you might choose to have it from time to time.

When you reach the end of your 30 day elimination diet, your system will be clear of any potential food triggers. At this stage you will probably notice some significant changes to your general health, your pain and stiffness, and your energy levels. The changes might be subtly pleasant or they may be dramatic improvements. It is at this time that you can begin reintroducing foods into your diet to see if they have any ill effects on you.

When re-introducing foods into your diet, follow these tips to ensure maximum accuracy:

1.) Introduce foods back into your diet one at a time with 3 to 5 days between each test. A reaction from a dietary trigger could happen immediately or take a few days to become apparent.

2.) Begin with the least offensive foods. For gluten, start with an unleavened bread or crackers rather than eating large amounts of bread. For dairy, try a drop of milk in your tea or coffee rather than a cheese or ice cream.

3.) Test with small amounts of possible triggers to avoid major set backs and unnecessary pain.

4.) Keep a diary showing when you are testing which foods to avoid mistakes.

5.) Be meticulous when analyzing your health. Write down any pain, stiffness, or discomfort. Take notes of any stomach upsets, headaches, or fatigue. Write down anything else you think may be significant.

Note: Everyone is different. You may find that some food gives you very mild discomfort whereas others may seem like they've caused a major flare-up. You know your body best so always trust your gut instinct and do what's right for you.

6.) If you have had a negative reaction to a food, avoid eating it again. Leave a few extra days before trying the next one to give your body time to relax and readjust.

7.) If you find that you have no reaction to something, be sure to introduce it back into your system slowly over a few days or weeks rather than bingeing on it.

As I have stressed a number of times in this book, everyone is different. Certain things about your story will be similar to other people's stories but remember that when it comes to your condition, you're the boss. Listen to your body and trust your own perceptions. For me, in my journey, I noticed that within the first two weeks of my elimination diet I was no longer taking painkillers or anti-inflammatories. My joints felt looser, I was much more agile, and for the first time in years I had multiple pain-free days under my belt. In addition, I was sleeping much better, my energy levels were up, and my mood was great. I was feeling positive and *healthy* for the first time in years! At my next visit to the doctor, I found out that my vitamin levels were all in the normal range and the inflammation in my blood was at an all time low. But the most significant changes were still to come. Because next, I started increasing my intake of beneficial foods and that's when things starting getting really good.

Step Three: Get Into The Good Stuff!

Although an elimination diet can do worlds for your understanding of your condition and it can make a huge difference to your daily aches and pains, you can make even more of a difference by making sure you're getting as many beneficial foods into your diet as possible. Plus learning about cooking new ingredients and optimizing the health benefits of your meals can be interesting and fun.

There are a large variety of vitamin rich foods that contain naturally occurring anti-inflammatory properties. Getting these foods in your daily diet in addition to taking some of the supplements I discussed earlier could make the difference between feeling good and feeling great! This next list will show you just how many foods have the power to ensure optimum health and keep your arthritis at bay.

1.) Cruciferous Vegetables
These vegetables are the ones your parents probably encouraged you to eat as a child so you would grow up to be big and strong! And guess what, your parents were right! Cruciferous vegetables include broccoli, brussel sprouts, cabbage, cauliflower, kale, chard, collards, and other dark greens. These veggies are packed with vitamins, nutrients, and fiber; all of which are very beneficial to your overall health. Cruciferous vegetables also include antioxidants, calcium, and B vitamins; all of which are vital nutrients in the fight against arthritis. Most importantly, cruciferous vegetables are packed with vitamin C which supports the immune system and helps the body make collagen, aiding joint flexibility and preventing further joint damage.

2.) Sweet Potatoes
In addition to their antioxidant properties, these delicious alternatives to white potatoes are brimming with beta carotene; a powerful weapon against inflammation and inflammatory conditions including OA and RA. They are also a very versatile vegetable that can be used in anything from curry to stews to a healthier version of french fries!

3.) Avocados

Avocados contain antioxidants, essential fatty acids, and vitamin E; all of which can aid the repair of cartilage meaning less inflammation and significantly reduced pain from both OA and RA. In addition, avocados can prevent further inflammation and damage to connective tissue. Getting these delicious, creamy fruits into your diet could prevent the need for painkillers and anti-inflammatory drugs. I suggest adding avocados to salads, smoothies, burritos, sandwiches, or as a simple topping for toast or crackers.

4.) Olive Oil

Unlike animal fats, hydrogenated fats, and many vegetable oils, olive oil can have a positive effect on arthritis and other illnesses. Olive oil contains mono-unsaturated healthy fats which help reduce inflammation, move healthy nutrients into the body's cells, and remove waste product. Using olive oil instead of other cooking oils is an easy way to give your body a little extra help fighting your condition.

5.) Ginger

Ginger contains both naturally occurring anti-inflammatories and salicylic acid which can ease pain and discomfort. It is available in a number different forms including raw, ground, oil, extract, and capsules so there are many ways you can get it into your daily life. I like adding fresh ginger to stir fries, juices, granola, baked goods, and homemade teas!

6.) Green Tea

Green tea has been used medicinally in many cultures for centuries. It contains powerful anti-oxidants which could have a significant effect on inflammatory conditions including RA. In addition, a few cups of green tea each day could reduce your risk of other serious illnesses including cancer and heart disease. If you're not a big fan of green tea, you can find a number of different infusions in most grocery stores including green tea with mint, ginger, lemon, and more. Alternatively, add a squeeze of lemon and a drop of honey to liven it up! If you really can't stomach green tea but you still want its benefits, supplements are also available.

7.) Whole grains

The big difference between whole grains and processed white varieties of grains is that whole grain (including wheat, oats, rice, bulgar, buckwheat, etc) still contains their hulls which is where the most nutrients are found. Switching to whole grain breads, pastas, rices, and other grains is also a great way to control your weight as they contain longer lasting energies and keep you full for longer. Keeping your weight down can make a huge difference to your daily pain levels as weight reduction takes strain off your weight-bearing joints, aids mobility, and helps you sleep better at night. Whole grain varieties of your favorite foods tend to have a richer, more robust flavor too! Just make sure to follow cooking instructions, as whole grains usually require slightly longer cooking than white varieties.

8.) Cherries

Research has shown that cherries (and cherry juice) could reduce pain better than drug treatment in people suffering from OA, RA, and a variety of other joint conditions. Cherries are rich in antioxidants which can help prevent damage to the body's cells caused by free-radicals. They also contain naturally occurring anthocyanin that can reduce pain more efficiently than common anti-inflammatory drugs without causing stomach upsets. And the benefit of cherries doesn't stop there! They can also help headaches, sports injuries, gallbladder and kidney problems, tooth decay, and gout.

9.) Turmeric

This spice is often found in Indian dishes and has been used medicinally in both Indian and Chinese medicine to treat arthritis, bursitis, and digestive problems. Studies have shown that turmeric not only contains anti-inflammatory properties but it may also modify immune system responses. It is therefore, effective in people suffering with both OA and RA. Turmeric is available in capsule form and in its powder form can be added to curry and many types of rice dishes. You can also add it to smoothies or make a special tea by adding a teaspoon of turmeric to 500mls hot water with a squeeze of lemon, some freshly grated ginger, and a teaspoon of honey.

10.) Aloe vera

Aloe vera contains a large variety of nutrients which are beneficial to sufferers of all types of arthritis and other inflammatory conditions. These include vitamins A, B, C, and E, as well as the naturally occurring steroids bradykinin and salicylate. Aloe vera also contains glucosamine, a compound naturally found in cartilage. This means it can reduce inflammation and pain as well as repairing joint damage. Aloe vera is also very versatile. It can be taken orally as a drink or capsule, or used as a gel rubbed directly on sore joints and muscles.

11.) Astaxanthin
This newly discovered "super nutrient" is thought to be the most powerful known antioxidant on earth. Although part of the carotenoid family, astaxanthin is far more powerful than the 700 others in its class including beta-carotene. Produced in microalgea and consumed by fish and other sea creatures, astaxanthin can protect your cells, organs, and body tissues from inflammation and damage caused by free radicals and other toxins. It also goes further than other carotenoids, protecting your eyes, brain, and central nervous system. And of course, it significantly decreases inflammation which makes it useful in both preventing and treating rheumatoid arthritis, as well as injuries and damage to joints such as OA, repetitive strain, and carpal tunnel syndrome. Both shellfish and vegetarian supplements of astaxanthin are available; however, beware synthetic versions as they may not have the desired effect.

12.) Probiotics
You may have noticed that these days that there's quite a buzz about the benefits of probiotics, or "good bacteria". These bacterias which are normally present in the body, have a large array of health benefits including keeping common illnesses at bay, contributing to a healthy digestive tract, aiding weight control, fighting fatigue, menstrual symptoms, relieving joint inflammation, and many more.

There are a number of things that could deplete your body's natural supply of "good bacteria" including age, stress, hormonal and steroidal medications, excessive caffeine consumption, poor dietary habits, environmental toxins, and antibiotics. But for people suffering from inflammation of any type - especially RA and psoriatic arthritis - recent studies show a that low levels of probiotics in the body could be a serious contributing factor.

The theory behind this thinking is that having an irritated small intestine - which could be caused by certain medications, stress, or even a simple stomach bug - could cause "leaky gut" syndrome, a condition I mentioned earlier. This is a condition wherein food substances "leak" through the intestine and into the blood stream. Now, you may be wondering how having a "leaky gut" could possibly affect your joints. The answer is slightly complicated but quite intriguing. When food particles enter the blood stream, the immune system kicks into high gear in order to fight off these foreign particles. If you are already predisposed to joint pain and inflammation - most notably if you suffer from an autoimmune condition - your immune system could basically be "confused" about what it's fighting, and attack you body's healthy cells. If this is the case, you will likely experience an increase to your pain and inflammation.

This new way of thinking may seem a little "out there" but as more and more studies are conducted, it's becoming quite a popular thought. If you imagine that the problem does not lie in your joints at all but rather, your *gut*, it's more than possible that by taking regular amounts gut-irritating painkillers and medicinal anti-inflammatories, you could be causing yourself even *more* pain. And on top of that, your diet could be contributing to your pain as well! A diet rich in alcohol, unhealthy snacks, and simple carbohydrates can also lead to leaky gut.

So, how do you know if your joint condition is actually being caused or exacerbated by a problem in your gut? Have a look at the following list of signs and symptoms to see if your gut may need a little TLC.

Signs Of "Leaky Gut":
1.) Allergies such as hay fever and asthma
2.) Food allergies and/or intolerances
3.) Regular bouts of stomach upset and digestive problems
4.) Hormone disruption such as PMS

5.) Stress, anxiety, and depression
6.) Autoimmune conditions
7.) Chronic fatigue
8.) Chronic aches and pain such as arthritis and fibromyalgia

If you think you might have a "leaky gut", have no fear! There are ways to repair and restore your digestive system naturally, and doing so could make a huge difference to your joint pain. For best results, speak to a doctor or specialist who can guide you through the process. Remember to always consult your doctor before making any major changes to your diet, lifestyle, or medications.

Here's a few very basic steps you can take to keep your gut healthy:

1.) Get rid of the bad guys: Remove unhealthy foods and alcohol from your diet. If your stomach is being irritated by a medication, talk to your doctor about switching to an alternative one which may cause you less irritation. Make sure to take *all* your medications and supplements into account.

2.) Add helpful digestive aids: Talk to your doctor about taking some healthy digestive constituents such as digestive enzymes or hydrochloric acid to help ease the disturbance in your gut.

3.) Add probiotics: Rebuild colonies of probiotics, as well as prebiotics, to get your gut back to good health. There are literally *trillions* of strains of probiotics and ensuring that you're getting a few different types could help the process. Probiotics are found in "active" yoghurts as well as specially fermented food and drinks. Alternatively, you can get your probiotic levels up by taking oral supplements, mixing probiotic powder into drinks and smoothies, or even buying probiotic mints!

4.) Keep it up: Once your gut health is restored, reduce the risk of further digestive troubles by maintaining a healthy diet, getting plenty of exercise, and keeping stress levels at a minimum.

You may be surprised to find just how much your diet affects your condition and believe me, I know that it can be very difficult to make such significant changes to your lifestyle. All I can say is that, it does get easier. For me, the more positive results I achieved, the more excited I was to keep going. It was my goal to do everything and anything I could do to reclaim my life. And now that I feel so good, I wouldn't even consider eating the foods that were causing me so much pain and disruption. I made a choice: I would rather live without certain foods than live with my condition the way it once was.

Your journey is specific to you and your goals may be different to mine. But, as I'm sure you've seen so far, there are tons of things you can do to make living with your condition easier; from the effortless to the diligent.

Here's another short recap of how I used diet to reduce my pain and regain full body wellness:

1.) I detoxed my system
By flushing toxins out of my body through a cleansing diet and increased relaxation, I put my body back to "square one" so I could more easily see what foods were aggravating my arthritis. I drank plenty of water and significantly increased my intake of fruits and vegetables.

2.) I eliminated all possible triggers
In order to know exactly what foods were bothering me, I embarked on a 30 day elimination diet. I eliminated all possible dietary triggers. During this process I found that my pain had reduced significantly and my energy had increased.

3.) I slowly reintroduced foods back into my diet
One by one, I tried each possible food trigger to see if it had an effect on me. I kept a diary to ensure optimum accuracy and left a few days between each test. If I found that a certain food had any ill effect on my body, I stopped eating it and let my body relax and readjust before trying another food.

4.) I began eating more beneficial foods

In order to obtain optimum health, I began eating foods that are known to help with inflammation and joint pain. I treated my gut with probiotics to reduce the impact of any possible symptoms of "leaky gut" syndrome.

Exercising For Optimum Health

Exercise can be difficult for arthritis sufferers. Pain, stiffness, limited mobility, and fatigue can act as major obstacles where movement is concerned. Many arthritis sufferers worry that exercise is going to cause them further pain or injury because of their arthritis, so they give up things they love like sports, yoga, knitting, or hiking. Many of us also live with loved ones who insist on keeping us immobile, however good their intensions are! Your partner, friends, family, or children might insist on doing everything for you. They might insist that you rest constantly because you're going to "hurt" yourself if you try to move more or do things for yourself. This is can be a double-edged sword at times. It is wonderful and important to have people around to offer help when you need it but if your caregivers are overbearing and won't let you get out of bed, you can bet that your condition is not going to improve.

Having arthritis is not a reason to stop moving! In fact, quite the opposite is true. Getting regular exercise can do worlds for your condition. Arthritic and injured joints need exercise in order to heal. Getting the right kinds of exercise can improve mobility and reduce daily pain and stiffness dramatically. The important thing is to find a form (or a few forms) of exercise that suit your condition, your interests, and your life.

For me, I started by simply starting to walk more. I noticed that walking for twenty minutes in the morning really loosened up my joints and helped my mobility for the rest of the day. When I reached a stage where my pain was significantly reduced from my diet I started upping the ante. Little by little I added more exercise into my life. I started taking some of the exercise classes that I used to love before I got sick and found that my body was capable of a lot more than I thought. Also, the more regularly I exercised, the more capable of it I became. I had to rebuild my agility and stamina. You can imagine how hard it might be to get started on an exercise regimen if you've had months or even years go by without moving more than just getting around the house! But don't let yourself worry about that. Set realistic goals and take it slowly. Remember that the aim is to regain mobility, *not* to push yourself too hard and end up hurting yourself!

Before embarking on a new exercise regimen, always consult your doctor. The first few weeks of exercise can cause a little discomfort or an increase to your stiffness but this very common and the benefits in the future will well outweigh your early adjustment period. So what's the best type of exercise for people living with arthritis? The following list will show you the three most effective types of exercise arthritis sufferers can use to regain strength and mobility as well as to prevent further joint damage.

What Exercises You Should Do

1.) Cardio
Cardio - or aerobic - exercise is paramount to keeping a healthy cardiovascular system. If you move for 30 consecutive minutes 4 to 7 days per week your pain levels should be reduced considerably. The way cardio works is quite interesting because aerobic exercise affects both mind and body wellness.

Regular cardio exercise makes your heart beat more efficiently. When you are exercising your heart pumps more blood and increases the amount of oxygen being carried by red blood cells. If you exercise regularly, your heart won't have to work as hard when you're resting. Furthermore, the blood traveling to your brain is more heavily oxygenated. This, combined with an increase to endorphin levels can have a fantastic impact on your mood and mental wellbeing. It can help you cope with stress and alleviate emotional tension. Also, as I mentioned earlier, muscle wasting is a very serious concern for people living with RA. As the heart is a muscle, it too can waste away. Getting regular cardio workouts means strengthening the heart muscle and possibly extending your life.

Cardio workouts range from simple to intense and include things like walking, dancing, running, cycling, swimming, aerobics (including aqua-aerobics), and anything else that gets your heart beating faster. When choosing what type of cardio will suit you, choose something realistic and enjoyable. If you haven't been able to get out of bed for weeks, start by simply walking more or choose a low impact exercise class like aqua-aerobics. If you are already quite mobile, step it up by taking on regular cardio workouts a few times per week for optimum health and mobility.

If you have a particularly bad joint, choose a form of exercise that isn't going to cause it further injury. For instance, if your knee is bad, running probably won't be a great option for you! If your shoulder is bad, heavy weightlifting might not be great idea! For anyone starting a new work out regimen, it's important to start small. Doing too much too soon could cause injury or make you never want to exercise again! Begin by doing something that is a little challenging but not too hard. Choose a form of exercise that you already enjoy or try something new and see how you find it. The more you exercise you'll notice that your body will be able to do more and more. Your stiffness will loosen up and your overall wellness will increase. After two or three weeks, you'll be surprised at how different you feel and how much more you're capable of!

2.) Stretching

Flexibility is a key factor in mobility. Not only does it increase the range of motion in your limbs and spine, but it also decreases risk of injury. You know by now that over-resting your body can increase your pain and lower your mobility, but over-resting can also decrease your flexibility. This means that if you have a bad back and you rest it too much, your spine and hips will become less flexible and more pressure will be placed on your joints and tendons, therefore increasing your risk of further injury and pain.

You may have noticed that resting too much can make your muscles feel tight. When you get out of bed you may hobble or limp for a while before you can walk upright. This is because, as your body remains static, your muscles are effectively becoming shorter. When you stretch regularly you are elongating your muscles, giving them a wider range of motion. If you trip or fall while your muscles are short and tight, you're far more likely to injure yourself than if your muscles are supple from regular stretching.

Stretching is a very versatile form of exercise that can fit into anyone's lifestyle. You can do it at home or at the gym. You can stretch with a physiotherapist or alone. Doing stretches in a warm bath or a hot tub can help to soften the muscles and connective tissue with less impact. Stretching classes such as Pilates, tai chi, and yoga can be very beneficial to people with arthritis and back pain. These practices focus a lot of attention on your "core" muscles; those found in your abdominals and your back. Core muscles are responsible stabilizing the body and absorbing movements in the limbs. For instance, imagine kicking your leg as high as you can. Even if your leg muscles are flexible, if your core muscles are weak, you could end up falling or twisting in a way that could cause a serious injury.

Regular stretching and strengthening your core muscles also increases balance; another key point in mobility and safety. It is common for people with RA and other autoimmune conditions to experience clumsiness and loss of balance. This aspect of the disease can be very unsettling, not to mention risky. Getting involved with something like tai chi or yoga can be a very helpful where balance is concerned.

3.) Resistance Training
Resistance training is an important way to prevent and treat muscle wasting; a process where the body loses muscle mass and strength. There are a number of things that can cause muscle wasting including age, diet, and (you guessed it!) arthritis! It's important to do what you can to prevent muscle wasting and rebuild strength where muscle loss is affecting your body.

Arthritis sufferers often experience muscle wasting due to not using their muscles enough (usually because their pain and stiffness causes discomfort). The problem here is that the less you use your muscles, the less strength you will have. And the less strength you have, the less mobile you will be *and* the more discomfort you'll feel when going about your daily life.

The good news is that rebuilding muscle mass and preventing muscle wasting is pretty straight forward. Resistance training is exercise that's designed specifically for muscle development. Weightlifting is the most common type of resistance training. Depending on your age and the specifics of your condition, you might not be able to get involved with heavy weightlifting but even lifting very light weights can help increase muscle mass significantly. If weightlifting is not for you, luckily, there are a number of other exercises that can help you keep your muscles at their best.

The most commonly wasted muscles in arthritis sufferers are those in the hands and thighs. This is why many people living with arthritis have limited dexterity and often experience feelings of exhaustion in their legs (even when they haven't done any exercise). There are many tools on the market nowadays that are specifically designed to strengthen the muscles in your hands. These are good because of their versatility. They can be used pretty much anytime and anywhere! Other exercises that can help with muscle wastage include cycling, climbing, using exercise bands with or without a physiotherapist, and doing simple at-home exercise like leg lifts and push ups.

The important thing to remember about preventing and treating muscle loss is that you will achieve the greatest results by coupling your exercise regimen with a healthy diet and a good sleep pattern.

I can't stress enough that in order to maintain strength, agility, mobility, and muscle mass, you simply have to move more. As I've mentioned earlier in this book, resting too much will decrease your mobility over time. Rest is important, but if you're going to be in charge of your arthritis - rather than letting your arthritis be in charge of you - you'll need to challenge yourself where movement is concerned. Remember to always stay safe when exercising and ask your physician if you have any concerns.

8 Great Exercises For People With Arthritis

Aquatic
Water is a fantastic medium for low-impact exercise. This is especially true when the water's warm, ranging between 83 and 88 degrees Fahrenheit (28.3 to 31.1 degrees Celsius). Submerging the body in warm water increases the body's temperature, which also increases circulation. One of the reasons water provides a healthy place to exercise is its buoyancy removes much of the weight off your joints and muscles. Water also adds resistance for your extremities, helping build strength. Water exercise options include swimming laps, walking in place in deep water or water aerobics classes. Hot tubs can also be therapeutic ways to massage aggravated muscles and relax after a workout.

Walking
Walking is the most accessible form of exercise for those with arthritis. All you have to do is open the front door and take the first step. Classified as a weight-bearing exercise, walking helps reinforce bone density by placing your full bodyweight on top of your bones and joints. It also strengthens your heart, lungs and overall endurance.
Start at a pace that will make you short of breath, but still able to talk. After a couple of weeks, increase the distance and pace. And I really recommend that you buy a pair of supportive sneakers.

Resistance Training
The gym can be a fun and inspiring place to exercise, no matter how old or young you are. There you'll find all the equipment necessary for strength and resistance training. This form of physical activity uses weight machines, free weights and resistance bands or tubing to strengthen muscles, bones, lungs and the heart. Resistance training has the ability to improve muscle strength, physical functioning and pain in 50 to 75 percent of people suffering from osteoarthritis of the knee.

There are two types of strengthening exercises: isometric and isotonic. Isometric exercise involves contracting the muscle without moving the joint, and it's particularly helpful if a certain joint lacks the ability to move. Isotonic exercise fortifies the muscle by moving the joint.

Tai Chi

Tai chi is a Chinese system of exercises that dates back thousands of years. It is practiced through a series of slow moving poses originally designed for self defense and mental calm and lucidity through its graceful circular movements and breathing techniques. Though the effects of tai chi lack much scientific study, it is believed to increase flexibility, strengthen muscles, develop balance and improve range of motion.

There are other reasons for people with arthritis to practice tai chi, including because it's low impact, has a low risk of injury and can be done indoors or outdoors, depending on your mood. It can also be practiced alone or in groups.

Yoga

Also an ancient form of exercise, yoga literally means to unite or yoke. The practice unites movement and breath and can help ease stiffness and tension in muscles and joints. However, you should be careful as some yoga moves could do you more harm than good. Getting into yoga does not have to mean joining a club – it can mean taking ten minutes by yourself at home everyday. An excellent book for getting started in yoga is "Yoga as Medicine" by Timothy McCall.

Cycling: Stationary or Outdoors

Biking is a great way to feel the wind in your hair and at the same time get in a low-impact aerobic exercise that improves the strength of your heart, hips and knees. And cycling can be done indoors in the winter months on a stationary bike, or outdoors when the air is warm and inviting. If cycling is new to you, start with short time slots of at least 10 minutes. Then extend those as your stamina improves.

Jogging

Just because you've been diagnosed with arthritis doesn't mean running is necessarily off your list of exercise activities! First you'll need a good pair of sneakers and perhaps orthotics to accompany them. Next, find a place to jog where the surface is flat and relatively soft. One option is to head to your local high school during their off hours and use the track. Not only will the surface give a little when you run, it also won't have the cracks, holes or debris that sidewalks or roads tend to have. Also, do remember to incorporate stretching into your jogging routine to prevent injury.

Personal Trainer or Physical Therapist

When it comes to exercise, if your get up and go has left the building, it may be best to turn to a trained professional to help restore your motivation. A personal trainer or physical therapist will help ensure that your exercise routine involves strength and endurance, flexibility and range of motion. These three facets of exercise are vital for helping ease and improve the symptoms of arthritis.

When choosing a professional to design your exercise program, find someone who'll be considerate of the fact that:

* People with arthritis are frequently less active
* Their range of motion is limited by swelling, pain and stiffness
* Repetitive movements can become painful after time
* Extra support and encouragement goes a long way

Your Mindset & How Much This Can Improve Your Pain!

I have mentioned the importance of maintaining a positive mental attitude throughout this book for many reasons. Scientific evidence has proven that there is a very strong connection between the mind and the body where health is concerned. If either your mind or body is suffering in some way, the other is likely to follow. This can be especially difficult when dealing with chronic and degenerative illnesses. Watching your mobility change over time can be very distressing. Feeling as though you cannot do the things you love or having a flare up when you are least prepared for it is one of the hardest things about living with arthritis. You may often feel frustrated and disheartened. Fears about the future can invade your thoughts and make you feel as if you have no control over your life. The unpredictability of inflammatory conditions can make it hard to work or even make simple plans. As your condition progresses and your life becomes gradually altered by it, your stress levels may rise. If you can't work anymore, you may experience added stress about money or you may grieve the loss of your passion or career path. If you're still quite young when these changes take place, you may experience even further upset! And as if all of that isn't hard enough to deal with - stress, depression, and anxiety can cause an *increase* to physical pain and poor health! It's a vicious cycle that can really get the better of you if you're not careful.

If allowed to, feelings of defeat and hopelessness can hold on to you like a vice, and the tighter that vice gets, the more your pain will increase and the less able you'll be to cope with it. Stress and negative thinking has been proven to have a negative effect on inflammation; causing more flare ups and increased difficulty recovering from them. Furthermore, when you're in a depressive state, you're less likely to care for yourself properly. You might not eat right. You might lose sleep. You're less likely to get fresh air and exercise. You may turn to alcohol or other substances to help with your pain. These things can make your energy levels plummet, and not only will your pain get worse from the lack of physical care, but taking poor care of yourself also sends a message to your body telling it to give up. This is why positive thinking and being optimistic are so important for arthritis sufferers.

Research has shown that people who exhibit a "fighting spirit" tend to live longer. They cope better with pain and serious illnesses and their bodies heal faster. In arthritis patients, an optimistic outlook has proven to reduce pain, making it possible to reduce the amount of pain killers and anti-inflammatories needed and increase mobility. Keeping your thoughts away from unhelpful ruminating is a powerful tool against pain. Wellness of the mind leads to wellness of the body so when you're embarking on your new natural treatment plan, it's important to make sure you include a care plan for your mind as well.

So what can you do to keep your spirits high? The next list offers you some important guidelines to help keep your thoughts on the positive tip.

Guidelines For Healthy Minds

1.) Don't worry about the future
Take each day as it comes. Worrying about the future will not change it. You will never know what your condition will be like in 10 years' time so obsessing over it is a waste of time and energy. Avoid making predictions about how your condition will be in the future. The future should be something you look forward to, not something you think about with dread. Trust that you are doing everything you can to keep yourself in good health and allow life to continue on its course.

2.) Don't let fear get the better of you
Courage is an important asset when living with any illness. If you require an operation or other procedure that you find anxiety provoking, it's important to remind yourself that fear will not change the situation. All fear does is make the situation more difficult to

cope with. To make things as easy as possible, practice acceptance and bravery where your condition is concerned.

3.) Only say things you KNOW are true
Often when we are nervous or anxious about something, our thoughts can spin a little out of control. We might indulge in a lot of "what ifs" or catastrophic thinking about situation at hand. This can be especially true during flare ups or times of extreme stress. Keeping your thoughts away from the worst case scenario can be difficult but it is a very important skill when it comes to positive thinking. A good way to slow down your racing thoughts is to only say (and think) what you know to be true. For instance, "today, my hands hurt" rather than "My hands might never get better... I won't be able to feed myself.... I'll need help for *everything*.", etc.

4.) Let go of things you cannot change
Don't allow yourself to spend time dwelling on things you can't change. Your condition will probably progress and change over time but it's important to remind yourself regularly that you are doing everything you can to improve your health and slow the progression of your illness down. Dwelling on things will not change the outcome; rather, it's likely to cause a dip in your mood and might lead you into a spiral of unhelpful thinking. Use your thoughts wisely by thinking of things you *can* do and things you *can* change. Let that be enough.

5.) Steer clear of internet forums
In this day and age people tend to dump their negative experiences on other people a lot. Whether it's a stranger online or a friend in the same room as you, if someone insists on telling you a horror story about *their* condition, don't let yourself get caught up in the drama and start overthinking *your* condition. Remind yourself that what someone else is sharing isn't *your* story. Your experience is autonomous. It is unique to you. Whatever happens to other people has no bearing on what will happen to you. Negative thinking is contagious! Make a resolve to try to turn negative conversations into positive ones or try to avoid them altogether.

6.) Think of the things you CAN do

Don't allow yourself to indulge in patterns of negative self talk. Negative thoughts are almost always based on emotions rather than facts. They may involve things at home, at work, or in your social life and they usually begin with "I can't". Reminding yourself of things you "can't" do can be depressing, and at its worse, it can prevent you from doing things you actually *can* do. Steer your thoughts away from negative tendencies by thinking and speaking in facts; i.e. "Today, I can do…". This will also help you deal with negative conversations. Often, your friends or relatives care so much about you that they thrust pity on you. This might lead them to insist on doing everything for you or it might mean that they say things that are unintentionally harmful to you. Having other people say how sorry they are for you about all the things you *can't* do, can really play tricks on your mind. They more someone says you can't do something, the more you'll start to believe it. Try to turn these conversations into positive ones by simply stressing the things you *can* do.

7.) Learn to let go and move on
Everyone has a tendency to feel sorry for themselves now and again and that's only natural. It can be hard to let go of things that you used to do and the way things used to be, but thinking too much about the past can be like beating yourself up with a stick. Do your best to try to let go of those things you lost and try to move on to new things that you might love just as much.

8.) Meditate
Meditation is a wonderful practice because it teaches you to quiet your dizzying thoughts and exist in the here and now. You can meditate absolutely anywhere and there are many different methods you can try. You can take guided meditation classes or stay in the privacy of your own home and listen to an audio cd. Just remember that meditation is called a "practice" because it takes practice! You won't be able to clear your mind of all thoughts right at the start but eventually you will learn how quiet them and feel good about life in the present.

9.) Avoid identifying as being "sick"

You are not your condition. Identifying as being sick sends a negative message to your body and eventually you will believe you can't do anything to improve your condition even when you can. As I mentioned earlier, when my RA was at its worst, it became a large part of my identity. I didn't notice it happening at first. I was so caught up in it all that it was all I thought about. I was blindsided by RA and I couldn't help but notice how much my body was changing and how much pain I was in. But the more I thought about being "sick", the worse I felt. Remember that you are much more than your condition. **Don't let arthritis define you!**

10.) Stay active

Fresh air and exercise are extremely beneficial for both your mind and your body. Often, people with arthritis make too many excuses to stay at home or in bed. Challenge yourself to get out and move regularly. Go to a nice place near water or take a walk in a scenic location. By taking time to get outside and keep your body active, you will see an improvement in your mood, your sleep patterns, and your pain levels.

11.) Socialize

It's important to continue to socialize with friends and family rather than hiding out at home because you're not in the mood. Isolating yourself from your loved ones is one of the worst things you to your mind because it separates yourself from normality and can make you feel very lonely. This can have devastating effects to your mood and how you view yourself in the world. Making time to see other people and talk about things other than your health is a great way to free yourself from your troubles, recognize the lives of others, and make you feel like you have people on your side.

12.) Be proud

As you embark on your journey toward wellness, be proud of yourself! You should feel good about what you're doing to make your condition better. Taking action that has a positive effect on your condition takes bravery and perseverance. Feel good about the commitment you've made to take charge of your pain! Give yourself a pat on the back when you push yourself outside your comfort zone and praise yourself for overcoming things you find difficult.

13.) Try something new

Living with arthritis often means giving up activities you love and that can be really hard to cope with. If you have lost the ability to do something you once enjoyed, don't give everything else up too! Think of your progressing condition as a means to try new things. Explore new interests and hobbies. Think about attending a class or a group that specializes in a hobby you might enjoy! Learning new things is a great way to stimulate brain function and keep your sights set on the things you *can* do rather than dwelling on the things you can't.

14.) Accept your condition

No matter how much you and your doctors do to make your condition easier to live with - even if you're able to put your condition in remission - it's very important for you to accept that (unless a cure is discovered) you will always have it. Some days will be harder than others and accepting that fact will help you cope better with unpredictable ups and downs. Making a commitment to treating your arthritis naturally should lead to plenty of pain free days and hopefully even years; however, when it comes to your emotions, it's important to have realistic expectations. Positive thinking can have wonderful effects on your pain, but more than anything, it should help you to cope with it better. Accepting your circumstances means that you're more likely to listen to your body. This way, if you're starting to feel like a flare up is coming, you're more likely to accept and prepare for it, rather than trying to fight it off and risk making it worse. This will lead to fewer disturbances in your life and a faster recovery while times are tough.

15.) Go easy on yourself

It's not possible to be "happy" all the time. It's important to recognize that having a positive mental attitude doesn't mean being perpetually happy. Everyone experiences difficult emotions. It's important to be kind and gentle toward yourself if you're feeling low. There's no point in beating yourself up. Remind yourself that what you're going through can be hard from time to time. Treat yourself the way you would treat a friend or loved one if they were in your position.

Before moving on to the concluding pages in this book, here's one final recap of the final part of my journey:

1.) I started moving more
In order to increase the benefits of my natural treatments, and start to enjoy my life again, I started doing small things to increase my daily movement. I began by taking short walks in the morning to help loosen up my joints. I started doing more things for myself rather than letting other people help me too much. I reminded myself that this part of my journey would be hard but that it would also be worth it.

2.) I began exercising regularly
When my mobility increased significantly, I started taking formal exercise classes to become even more mobile. I focused on cardio, stretching, and resistance training to regain strength and get my body as mobile as possible. I exercised at least 30 minutes each day as well as doing three rigorous exercise sessions per week.

3.) I focused on the present
I accepted my condition, stopped longing for the past, and avoided thinking about negative possibilities in my future. This way, I learned to enjoy life in the present and get the most out of life. I let go of fear and steered clear of negative thinking. I thought about the things I could do, rather than the things I couldn't do. I no longer identified as being sick and really started *living* again.

Escape The Pain & Live A Happy, Healthy Life

I hope that as you reach these last few pages, you are feeling uplifted and positive about your health and your future. I know first hand how difficult it can be to live with arthritis. On top of living with painful, stiff joints, your life can be greatly affected by your condition, causing limited mobility, loss of activities you once loved, increased stress levels, and sadness.

Discovering how to treat my RA naturally wasn't easy! It took a lot of hard work and dedication, but it was the best thing I have ever done. By taking the time to find out what was triggering my arthritis, I was able to eliminate harmful substances from my system and reduce both the regularity and severity of my flare-ups. By making changes to my diet and exercise regimes, I have become a healthier *and* happier person. My body is stronger and more capable than I ever thought it could be. I am no longer knocked down by common illnesses and injuries and I'm proud to say: have no problem keeping up with my children nowadays!

Whatever type of arthritis you have, it doesn't have to be the end of you. Whether you want to simply make things a little easier on yourself or you want to shoot for a full recovery is entirely up to you. You know your life and your condition better than anyone else. The bottom line is that there are things you can do to improve your condition and doing so can be greatly empowering! Your life is still your own! **If I did it, you can too!**

I wish you all the best on your journey.

Sarah Woodside

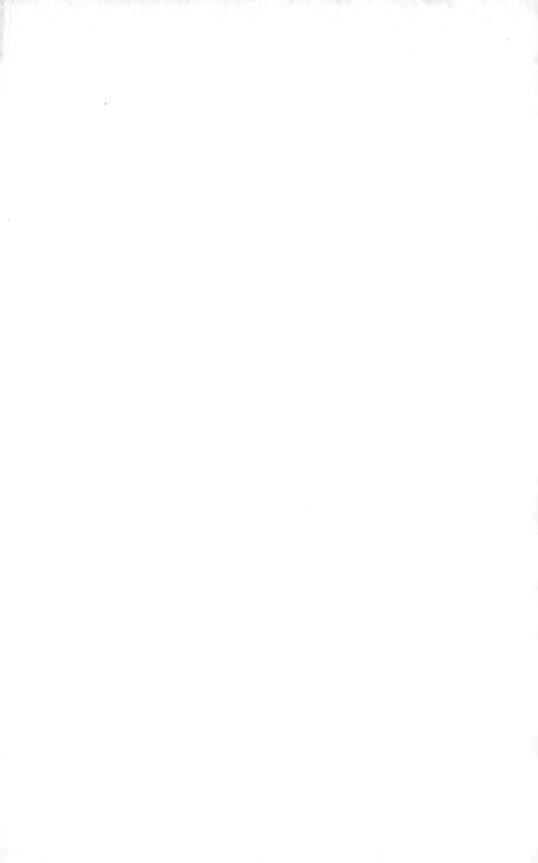

CPSIA information can be obtained
at www.ICGtesting.com
Printed in the USA
LVHW082238250119
605132LV00020BA/1015/P